Praise for *Facing Death*

"In *Facing Death*, Brad Stuart invites us to embrace the life force that underlies the deepest kinds of healing, whether in medicine or in our personal lives. Bringing together solid science, Eastern wisdom, and learnings from a lifetime of rich clinical practice, he invites us to embrace the awareness of our true nature. You can access this through meditation and altered states of consciousness today—or if you prefer to wait, it may surprise you at life's end. Clinicians may learn to blend curing and healing so they flow together, 'like two streams making a great river.' Anyone who reads this book will be prepared for transformative experiences in life's final moments—or in your life right now. You will not stop turning the pages of this brilliant book, and you will be glad you didn't."

— Dale G. Larson, PhD, McCarthy Professor, Counseling Psychology, Santa Clara University, author of *The Helper's Journey: Empathy, Compassion, and the Challenge of Caring* (2020 Research Press)

"The author has not just glimpsed, but experienced something that's very difficult to describe—yet he does a great job at describing it. He combines eastern and western mysticism and spirituality into a unified vision that our culture can really begin to grasp. In addition, he walks us to the edge of known science, then shines a bright light into the great mystery beyond. Blending nearly fifty years of medical practice with a deep dive into the healing value of meditation and psychedelics, this book presents a new paradigm for spiritual awakening."

— David S. White, Hospital Chaplain, author of *We Need to Talk: Conversations to Ease Fear and Suffering Surrounding End of Life* www.onemillionpledges.com

"In this book, Dr. Stuart reveals his own experiences with his greatest teachers – not professors of science or medicine, but his own patients. He weaves stories of his own involvement with LSD together with research on the benefits of psychedelics in serious illness, and his accounts of care of the dying with his own struggles with a cancer diagnosis. Brad has already made a profound impact on our field by developing new models of care for people with serious illness. But his spiritual insights may be even more important. He implores us to let go of what we as a society and as individuals tend to prioritize above all else—our *self*—throughout life, and most critically, at life's end."

> — Alex Smith, MD, MS, MPH, Professor of Medicine, University of California San Francisco and Co-host of the *GeriPal* podcast

"Thank you for this book and for guiding all your readers in understanding our oneness and our access to it. The writing is beautiful, intimate, clear, and even humorous. I felt like I was meditating the whole time I was reading."

> — Katharine Blank, RN, Labor and Delivery Nurse

FACING DEATH

Spirituality, Science, and Surrender at the End of Life

BRAD STUART MD

Capucia LLC
211 Pauline Drive #513
York, PA 17402
www.capuciapublishing.com
Send questions to: support@capuciapublishing.com

Paperback ISBN: 978-1-954920-65-1
eBook ISBN: 978-1-954920-66-8
Hardcover ISBN: 978-1-954920-67-5
Library of Congress Control Number: 2023905294

Cover Design: Ranilo Cabo
Layout: Ranilo Cabo
Editor and Proofreader: Karen Burton
Book Midwife: Karen Everitt

Printed in the United States of America

Capucia LLC is proud to be a part of the Tree Neutral® program. Tree Neutral offsets the number of trees consumed in the production and printing of this book by taking proactive steps such as planting trees in direct proportion to the number of trees used to print books. To learn more about Tree Neutral, please visit treeneutral.com.

Disclaimer

The purpose of this book is not to dispense medical advice or prescribe the use of any technique as a form of treatment for physical, emotional, or medical problems without the advice of a professional, either directly or indirectly. The intent of the author is to offer information of a general nature to help the reader in the quest for well-being. In the event the reader uses any of the information in this book for self or others, the author and the publisher assume no responsibility for the actions of the reader.

This book contains true stories and events. The author has shared these as accurately as memory will allow while acknowledging that memory is an imperfect recorder of history. In order to protect anonymity for persons both living and deceased, many names have been changed.

To Barbara, who knows

Contents

Introduction

When I entered medical school in the fall of 1974, the last thing on my mind was spiritual transformation. I was simply excited that I might learn how to cure disease. Little did I know that there's a big difference between curing and healing—and that medical training is all about curing. I would have to learn healing on my own.

I wasn't one of those kids who knew that I wanted to be a physician at age five. A career in medicine might not have occurred to me at all if it weren't for a remark from one of my college professors.

I was a senior working in Burt Weiss's physiology lab at Drexel University in Philadelphia. My job was to place tiny silver electrodes into the inner ears of tadpoles to study their hearing. Tadpoles live underwater, but like all amphibians, their anatomy and physiology—including their organs of hearing—change radically once they grow legs and move onto dry land.

Anyone who has read Carl Jung knows that frogs are a striking symbol of transformation. But that fact was totally lost on me.

I had started out in Chemical Engineering as a freshman in 1967, just as the Summer of Love erupted in San Francisco. I loved chemistry in high school, but chemical engineering took all the heart out of chemistry, and engineering had nothing to do with people—just things. So I dropped it, then cycled through several different majors, ending up in Humanities and Social Sciences.

Drexel is a five-year, work-study school, with the majority spent half in class and half out in industry. Knowing I wanted to move west someday, I landed a job with a ball bearing company and drove a Rambler American 30,000 miles in six months to visit every auto parts store west of the Mississippi River, or so it seemed. Sure enough, the day my Rambler rolled into the San Francisco Bay area, I knew I'd found my future home.

But first I had to graduate from college. I was interested in both clinical psychology and neurophysiology, but I couldn't visualize a career that would connect them. To be honest, I learned more from my extracurricular experiences with LSD and psilocybin than from most of the material presented in the classroom.

I had always sensed there was something beyond my little self. In high school, my idea of a hot date was to take my girlfriend out parking in the woods. Then we would stare together out the windshield of the car up at the stars. The universe was so immense, we were so small, and somehow that was just perfect. Then psychedelics blew a hole in the wall that had separated me from knowing that the universe consists of so much more than just the stars in the sky.

Graduation loomed, but I had no idea what I wanted to do next. Professor Burt was aware of my quandary. One day as we took a break, he gave me a piece of advice. "You should be a doctor," he said. "You like science, you're good with your hands, and you know how to get along with people."

That comment was a bolt of lightning out of a clear blue sky. It took me a second to pull my scattered wits back together. "Burt," I said finally. "You are out of your mind."

Burt and I published a paper about our work, and then I bid him a fond farewell. After graduation, I walked down the street to the University of Pennsylvania, pulled an index card off the *Help Wanted* bulletin board, and found my next job, again as a lab tech.

This time, I worked at the Johnson Research Foundation under the direction of Britton Chance, a brilliant biophysicist who narrowly missed winning a Nobel Prize for discovering how the body obtains energy as it passes electrons along a specialized chain of enzymes. Brit was a high achiever. In his hobby of sailing, he won an Olympic gold medal piloting a boat of his own design.

Brit's lab covered two floors of a large building on the Penn campus. The lab never closed—scientists from all over the world worked there twenty-four hours a day, seven days a week. The atmosphere crackled with excitement.

Brit was fond of designing intricate pieces of equipment and fabricating them in his own machine shop. But he was frustrated by his newest gizmo, designed to measure oxygen levels in rat brains through changes in reflected fluorescent light. "The damn thing just won't work," he complained. He hired me to make it operate properly.

It turned out that the machine worked fine, but nobody had been patient enough to anesthetize a lab rat, do some delicate surgery on it (you don't want to know the details), and keep it alive for hours while doing measurements on its brain.

The results were good—for the experiment, not for the rats. I took the data to Brit's photography and computer staff and developed a 3-D image of the surface of the brain in *normoxia*—while breathing room air—and *hypoxia*, when inspired oxygen levels were reduced. The effect of hypoxia on the human brain is profound, as every human experiences at the time of death. I had no way of knowing this in 1972.

Brit and I became friends. He had me over for Christmas dinner when he found out I wasn't going home; he was a father figure for me as I didn't have much of a relationship with my own dad. My father was a dour and intimidating person who taught me to hate religion, forbidding any mention of God in our household. Consequently, I never gave spirituality a thought. This probably magnified the impact of psychedelics on my brain a few years later.

One day Brit called me into his office. "It's time to publish our results," he said. "Go ahead and write the paper."

I didn't have the faintest idea how to write a scientific paper. Burt had written the one we'd published at Drexel. But after reading a few other papers and learning the language of biophysics, I produced a manuscript. Brit liked it. In fact, he thought it was good enough to submit without much revision.

It had been over a year since Professor Burt had made the outlandish suggestion that I should become a doctor. That's how long it took to get it through my head that I might make it in medicine.

The competition for the few sacred spots at top-level medical schools was fierce. As Brit and I sat in his office discussing the manuscript submission, I decided to take a gamble. "Brit," I said, "what would you think if we put my name first on this paper?"

That would be a serious tradition-breaker. I was a measly lab tech without any credentials. Brit, on the other hand, was internationally famous. His office walls were lined with piles of the articles he'd published. His secretary would walk in as we talked and pull copies off the stacks in response to requests for reprints from around the world. A paper with his name on it would be accepted immediately by any high-impact scientific journal.

Brit peered over the top of his reading glasses, squinting at me as he took a long pull on his pipe. "Oh, what the hell," he laughed. "Why not?"

Our paper was published. I made my first presentation at a national conference. I published several other papers that year, collaborating with friends from Israel, Australia, Japan, and many other countries.

I applied to just one medical school, a highly regarded institution in the San Francisco Bay area. My application must have raised a few eyebrows because I didn't get invited for an interview. As the deadline drew closer, I called the Office of Admissions and requested one. The receptionist put me on hold for an agonizing ten minutes, then came back on. She told me to show up the next Monday morning.

It was Thursday. I rushed around the lab and borrowed money from all my friends for a cross-country plane ticket and a night in a cheap hotel. I made the Sunday flight and marveled at the palm trees as I drove my rental car through the majestic campus. My interview was with the Chief of Chest Surgery. We hit it off immediately and talked for two hours.

All I remember about our conversation was that I supported paying for medical care for the poor. I regretted it later because that topic was just as controversial then as it is today. But I must not have blown the interview too badly. Soon after I returned to Philadelphia, a letter of acceptance arrived in my mailbox.

I packed all my belongings into my VW bus, drove to California, and found an apartment in Menlo Park over the Whole Earth Truck Store. After we started, my classmates and I were told that the admissions committee had decided to select *interesting students* that year.

I marveled at my good luck. The winds of fate had filled my sails and carried me to a whole new world.

The first two years of medical training were intoxicating. Our lecturers included seven Nobel laureates. They told us that science was only beginning to unravel secrets that would explain the fabulous intricacies of life. I thought I might become an eminent specialist, maybe a cardiologist. But fate had other ideas.

Part 1 of this book starts at the beginning of my third year, when medical students go on the wards to see patients. What I experienced there convinced me that we doctors have much more to learn than what science has to teach.

My mission changed. I stopped wanting to be a specialist. Instead, I wanted to learn as much as I could, not just about curing ordinary diseases, but about helping people heal—especially when their diseases can't be cured.

Beyond that, I wanted to help our health system heal. I had learned that in our rush to cure, we cause harm—and we don't even know it.

I finished my medical training as quickly as I could. Then I moved to a small town north of the Bay Area and practiced general internal medicine in my office, the emergency room, hospital, and ICU for over ten years.

It dawned on me that I was learning more from people who were dying than from those whose lives I saved. So I closed my practice and went into full-time end-of-life care. I started as a hospice medical director, initially at a small agency near my home in Sonoma County, California. That hospice merged with the largest not-for-profit healthcare system in Northern California, and I became senior medical director for home-based services in that system.

I got involved at the national level to improve care for people at the end of life. I led a team of doctors from around the country as we combed through the world literature on prognosis in non-cancer disease. We published a set of guidelines on estimating prognosis for the National Hospice Organization to help doctors know when people with heart failure, COPD, Alzheimer's, and others were ill enough to receive hospice services. Although we didn't employ advanced statistical methods to prove the accuracy of our predictions, more rigorous analysis with better data fifteen years later bore out most of our hunches.

Still, I watched many people enter home hospice with less than twenty-four hours to live, often straight out of the ICU. I thought the process might improve if we went upstream and brought care to seriously ill people at home before they were at death's door. I put a small team together, and we received a grant to create a program called Comprehensive Home-Based Options for Informed Consent about End-Stage Services (CHOICES).

The next step was to use home health, a service separate from hospice, to do the same thing. We gave this program a more streamlined title: Advanced Illness Management (AIM). In 2010, the Affordable Care Act (a.k.a. Obamacare) became law, creating the Centers for Medicare and Medicaid Innovation (CMMI). Congress appropriated $1 billion to fund Round One of CMMI's Health Care Innovation Awards.

Our team won a $13 million grant to spread AIM across our entire health system. After a two-year pilot, CMMI determined that AIM improved quality of care and reduced healthcare costs significantly. Medicare decided that a new source of financing should be developed to pay for home-based care like AIM. My team and I flew back and forth to Washington, DC, to advise CMMI as they determined how to do this. When the new payment models were implemented nationally in 2019, we were happy we had played a part in health system transformation.

When I made the transition from curative to end-of-life care, I didn't think much about what motivated that change. It was only after I spent enough time with people who were making their own transition to dying that the motivation became clearer.

That motivation was spiritual transformation. But just as *I* was in the dark about this for years, spiritual transformation may not be what *you* think it is. That's because most people who talk about spirituality put it in the context of living a meaningful and fulfilling life.

Living a meaningful life is as much about morality and ethics as it is about spirituality. If there's one thing I've learned from people at the end of life, it's that living a good life will be only a small part of what I'll be considering when I'm about to die. I will have let most of those earthly thoughts go, along with everything else I've done, possessed, felt, or thought.

At the moment I depart this life, I will be left with one thing only: *who I really am*. I came in with that, and I'll leave with that. The same goes for you.

I wrote this book to sum up what I've learned about all this over a long, eventful, and ultimately satisfying life—although it didn't always feel satisfying as it was happening. I had to learn some lessons the hard way, but gaining wisdom from these learning experiences is what we're here to do. This learning is not so much about accumulating knowledge as it is about knowing when to let go, to unlearn what you think you know.

Don't worry about packing for this trip that is your life. Before you get to your destination, you may have some serious unpacking to do.

Lest you think I'm trying to come across as some kind of spiritual authority, I need to insert a caveat: *He who gives advice is talking to himself.*

That statement has a couple of different meanings. First, be careful when you listen to anyone who wants you to buy their beliefs—especially when they involve the end of life or what may come after. Those beliefs may just be formulated to give comfort to the person who developed them and to generate support for their own system of thought.

That's not what Buddha, Jesus, or other great spiritual visionaries had in mind when they decided to take their message to the world. What they intended was to induce transformation in the hearts and minds of those who had ears to hear.

I don't intend to be a spiritual teacher or a religious leader, and I don't want any followers. Just read what's in here, take to heart what's useful to you in your search, and let go of the rest. That action will help prepare you for the ultimate spiritual practice: letting go of everything you think you know.

The second meaning is: I actually *am* talking to myself. Yes, I wrote this book for you, the reader, but I'm also talking to the you that was me: the younger, more confused, and disillusioned version of myself who lived fifty years ago.

I entered medical school in 1974 armed with experience in brain research, clinical psychology, psychedelics, and a sort of rudimentary spirituality that had nothing to do with religion. I was looking forward to medical education. Instead I received medical *training*—instruction in the technical aspects of curing disease.

What I was really looking for was *education* in the spiritual aspects of healing human beings. The word *education* has two different Latin roots. *Educare* pertains to *bringing up*, as in training a child. This has to do with applying layers of knowledge in the mind to succeed in the world. The other root word, *educere*, has more to do with *bringing out*, developing qualities that are already present in the individual in a nascent form. This process involves removing layers of knowledge from the mind to foster a personal relationship with the eternal.

Medical training needs to employ more bringing out and less bringing up. In other words, more emphasis on healing and less on curing— particularly for people near the end of life. Educere, bringing out, developing what's already within you—that's what this book is about.

But more fundamentally, this book is about *you*. Who are you? Are you the person you've worked hard to develop, so that you can be the best *self*—the most enlightened individual—you can be? If that's your aspiration, I wish you well, but that's not what I'm talking about.

One of the deepest spiritual truths is that the *self* you've worked hard to develop and the *you* who is your genuine essence are two different things. You may spend your whole life on the first one, only to arrive at the end of your life to discover that you've missed out on the second.

Fortunately, the real *you* is waiting to be discovered deep inside the *self* you think you are. It may be worthwhile to do some work to realize this. The work centers on letting go of the parts of your self that aren't really you—that's the unpacking. You may choose to postpone this work, but don't worry. Dying will do it for you. Either way, by the time you're ready to leave this place, all that will remain is the real *you*.

And to that younger version of myself: *I know I spent a lot of time and energy trying to be that special person.* My advice to that younger me is: *Don't stop there. Keep looking.*

Part I of this book is a collection of stories that illustrate my journey of learning through medical training and practice. I'm grateful to my medical teachers, even though I had trouble with some of their teachings. Luckily, my real teachers were the people I encountered in my work. Doctors tend to call them patients. That term sometimes makes me uncomfortable, because thinking of them as patients may encourage us to forget that they're people with human concerns that transcend the physical level we doctors are trained to focus on. But these folks were certainly patient with me as I learned from them. I'm more grateful than I can say.

Part II details spiritual insights that have dawned on me over these decades. When you work with people who are dying, it takes time to realize that most of the phenomena you think you're seeing, and most of the insights you think you're having, are products of your own experience, filtered through your own mind.

That's true of life in general. The world is a mirror that reflects your self, a product of your own mind, back to you. But if you follow life right out to its edge, you might begin to have inklings of what might lie beyond. Mystics have talked about this for thousands of years—perhaps today we finally have ears to hear.

Part III explores some of the implications of the thoughts expressed in Part II. How can you go beyond your own limited mind to experience, not merely fantasize about, what's ultimate and eternal—and bring this experience down to earth so it can be useful to you while you're still here? Although it's not widely appreciated, science and spirituality are coming together to show how some ancient tools work today. Research in meditation, psychedelics, and remembered experiences of death (RED) show that many people are already seeing through the mirror. The same fields of knowledge I brought to medicine—brain research, clinical psychology, and a more developed spirituality—are applied here.

If you're a skeptic, welcome to the club. I used to be skeptical too. We are all mystics. It's just that most of us don't know it yet.

Much of the material in this book is packed densely into the writing. I've tried to make it conversational and easy to read. You could probably forge straight through in one or two sittings. But to get the most out of your reading experience, I encourage you to bookmark sections that attract your attention, then go back and review them later.

And pay close attention to that attraction. The part of you that is attracted is the part of you that this book is all about.

It's easy to get discouraged these days. Our world is ever more complex and daunting. But now is not the time to give up. Instead, it's time to surrender outmoded concepts regarding your self and your world. Then buckle up. Our entire culture may be entering a revolution in our understanding of reality and a new paradigm in our spirituality and our science. You are hereby invited to participate.

So let's begin. *You are not who you think you are.* Regardless of whether you're a reader or you're me, that's a good place to start.

PART I

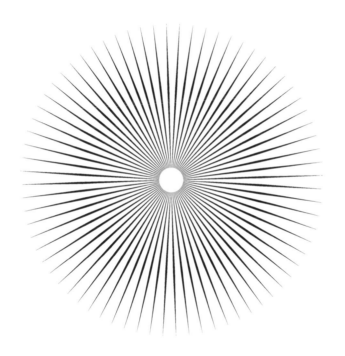

LEARNING

CHAPTER 1

Curing Versus Healing

Mr. Crawford lay silently in the darkened hospital room. The light hurt his eyes. His wife sat devotedly by his bedside.

The patient had a rare cancer of the immune system. In 1976, I was a third-year medical student. I was finished with the first two years of lectures and cadaver dissection. This was my first clinical rotation, and Mr. Crawford was my first patient.

I tried to take a history, but the patient could barely talk. I examined him, drew blood for labs, and started an IV. Most people flinch when they're stuck. He didn't. I felt like I should say something. I didn't.

The lab results showed his blood cell counts were near zero across the board. The Resident took a bone marrow sample. The marrow was packed with tumor, replacing nearly all the blood-forming elements.

Mr. Crawford was on a research protocol. He was set to receive a new form of chemotherapy that worked by wiping out nearly all the cells in his bone marrow. If he was lucky, normal cells would grow back before the cancer did. But Mr. Crawford had very few normal cells in his bone marrow.

It seemed to me this treatment would likely kill him. I mentioned my misgivings to the Resident. He reacted with scorn. "You don't get it," he said. "This place is Mecca. People fly here from all over the world when nothing else works. Get used to it."

The Resident's answer was accurate, but not satisfying. So I went up the food chain to the Chief Resident. He agreed to call a meeting to discuss the case. An hour later, the meeting room was packed with white coats.

The room fell silent as the Chief stood to speak. "Dr. Stuart has a few thoughts about the cutaneous T-cell lymphoma in 108."

He was being sarcastic. I wouldn't get my MD for at least two more years—if I made it that far. And he referred to the patient as a disease with a room number. It was irritating. I stood up and faced the crowd. In the front row sat the Dean of the medical school. I took a deep breath and started in. "This patient's disease is extremely advanced," I said. "If we do nothing, he will die. But if we treat him, he will probably die sooner. Should we really give this drug?"

Silence. Finally, the Dean spoke. "It's the only chance he has."

A chance somewhere between slim and none, I thought. But his response was understandable. Mr. Crawford and his wife were expecting him to be cured, or as close as he could get. The Resident was right—that was the business we were in. I had to move on. "There's another issue though," I said. "Shouldn't someone talk to him and his wife? They have no idea what they're dealing with."

Everyone looked down. It was like we were meeting to consider physician footwear. Finally someone spoke. "I don't believe we have a language for this."

I wanted to suggest, "How about English?" But I didn't.

It was strange that there was no response to that second question. The first question was about curing, and the second one was about healing.

Weren't we there to do both?

The meeting broke up. Ten minutes later, the Chief caught me in the hall. "They're going to treat him," he said.

"Okay," I said. "I'd like to give the medication myself."

The Chief examined me carefully, eyebrows raised. He was not going to make this easy.

"It's a learning experience," I said.

"Suit yourself," he replied over his shoulder as he walked back up the hall.

I knew I would never forget this day. Little did I know it would determine the direction of my career.

I mixed Mr. Crawford's medication myself and drew it up into a syringe. The drug was a vivid day-glow scarlet. I was holding a bolt from hell in my hand. I took the syringe to Mr. Crawford's room. Mrs. Crawford gazed at me with eager anticipation. "Here's your husband's medicine," I said.

"Thank God!" she exclaimed.

By this time, her husband was unconscious. I was dying to say something. But lack of training, and lack of courage, kept me silent.

In those days, there were no IV pumps. I connected the syringe to the port in the patient's IV line and depressed the plunger carefully. The crimson liquid flowed through the IV tubing into his vein. When the infusion was done, I said goodbye and left.

The next morning I went straight to Room 108. The patient's mattress was bare, the sheets stripped off the bed. I asked the Resident what had happened to Mr. Crawford.

It took him a moment to recall. "Oh yeah," he said. "He dropped his platelets to zero overnight, bled into his brain, and died."

I walked down the hall, fists and teeth clenched. That was certainly a *Learning Experience*—but not the kind I was expecting.

I couldn't help thinking of the lab animals I'd sacrificed in the quest for scientific knowledge. The way we had treated Mr. Crawford felt so similar that I could hardly bear the thought. It wasn't the last time I would see this kind of callous disregard for suffering play out in academic and community hospitals and ICUs.

I realized that my chosen profession of medicine had a serious problem. We had become desensitized to the suffering we caused. I had no religion, yet I felt we had committed both a sin of commission in deciding to treat the patient when we knew it would speed his death, and a sin of omission by deciding not to talk with him and his wife about the consequences of our actions.

We had both abused and neglected our patient, and we hadn't even realized it. And I was the agent who had done the deed.

We were not simply desensitized. In fact, a bigger problem was our hypersensitization. We were so sensitive about the end of life that we could not even acknowledge that it was a possibility. Because of our fear, we refused to face death.

Mr. Crawford and his wife had the same problem. Because they could not admit that death was coming, they had come to us asking for a miracle. We had agreed to their request because giving in to death would have amounted to failure.

We had conspired with the patient and his wife in a monstrous collective refusal to face death. And we were just as unconscious about this process as we were about the suffering we caused.

That made me think. *How would it look if we all summoned the courage to face death together?* The thought followed, *I've got to write a book about this.*

Immediately a loud voice replied. "You'll write your book," it said. "But only when you don't want to."

I looked around to see who had spoken. Nobody was there.

It was a Zen koan from nowhere.

Nearly half a century has passed since Mr. Crawford died. That's how long it took for these matters to settle themselves in my mind.

That voice was right. This is not the book I wanted to write that day. It's the one I needed to read that day.

I used to wish that voice had said more. Today, I'm thinking it might have said something like this: "You think your professors are wrong. But the mistake is also yours. You assume you know what death is. Think again."

CHAPTER 2

A Message from a Friend

After my first year in medical school, during the summer of 1975, I flew home to the East Coast. A friend in Baltimore asked me if I'd like to go with him and his wife to see a psychic. I was more of a believer in physics than in psychics, but I said yes.

I sat in Laurie's office, facing her on the other side of a small table. There were no Tarot cards or other props. She just talked. The first half hour was uneventful but intriguing. Somehow, without my saying more than hello, she seemed to know certain things about my personality.

Suddenly Laurie halted in mid-sentence and gazed at a point above my right shoulder. "Do you know someone named Cody?" she asked.

I had to stop and think. Then I remembered. "Oh yeah," I said. "Cody was a friend in high school."

How could I forget? Memories flooded back. I knew Cody from second grade on. He and I were both raised out in the country in Pennsylvania. We were on the high school track team together. I was a mediocre sprinter and long jumper. But starting at about age twelve, Cody went down to the creek by his place and cut young, tall, and straight black birch trees with trunks of just the right thickness to support his weight. Then he taught himself to pole vault.

In high school, they gave Cody a fiberglass pole. He immediately set records, then won a full scholarship to the University of Pennsylvania.

We both entered college in the fall of 1967. I went to Drexel, right up the street from Penn in West Philadelphia.

The tsunami released by the Summer of Love was washing over the East Coast as we entered our freshman year. The distractions were endless— the Vietnam War, the draft lottery, the King and Kennedy assassinations, the protests, the student strikes, and, of course, psychedelics.

I always treated these substances with respect, and they returned the favor. Years later, the insights I had gained early on from LSD and psilocybin would make major contributions to my work with people near the end of life. We'll talk about psychedelics and the mystical experience in more depth later. For now, we need to look at one central question they raise.

When you take a sufficient dose of LSD, your ego dissolves and you experience the bliss of knowing—not mere intellectual knowing, but absolute certainty—that all of reality is one living unity, it's all made of love, and it all emerges from a great void that is somehow supremely conscious.

Then you come down and you're back in yourself. It's monumentally irritating.

Here's the insight nobody seems to talk about. You experience your ego dissolving. You see ultimate reality. You come back to yourself.

The only constant through that whole experience is—*you*. The place inside that is simply aware.

That basic awareness that sees and experiences doesn't change at all, even when your self and your reality are blasted to smithereens. Then your world all pulls back together by itself as if the pieces are somehow magnetized. And the unchanging *you* witnessed the whole thing.

Which begs the question: Who are *you*?

I lost track of Cody for a few years until one day I met him on the street. He was dressed in white pants and a white shirt, with a round white paper hat on his head and a wispy beard. I asked him what he was up to.

"That's my ice cream truck over there," he said.

"Wow, that's great," I replied, trying to sound unsurprised. "How's it going at Penn? Are you still vaulting?"

"No, man," he said. "The classes, the track team—it was all way too intense. I dropped out."

"Seriously?" Now I couldn't conceal my shock. "How are you doing?"

His face fell a little before he replied. "I'm good. Making a living. Thinking of going back home though."

We enjoyed a big hug, and he walked back to his ice cream truck. That was the last time I ever saw him.

I later heard from Cody's family that he did return home. He turned his talents to music, learned to play the guitar, and started a band. He also got way into drugs.

I didn't mention any of this to Laurie. Which was fine. She didn't need any material from me.

"Cody's here with us right now," she said. "He has a message for you."

"Really?" I said. "What is it?"

Laurie replied, "He says no matter what you hear, don't worry. You need to know everything is fine."

"Strange," I said. "What does he mean by that?"

"I have no idea," said Laurie. "That's everything—nothing else is coming through."

The next day I drove up to see my parents in Pennsylvania. I walked in the front door carrying my suitcase. Before I could put it down, my mother ran up and thrust a newspaper clipping into my free hand. "You've got to read this," she said. "It just happened yesterday."

I put my suitcase down, gave her a hug, and read the clipping.

Cody ran his motorcycle at high speed into a tree and died—the day I had my reading with Laurie.

I thought a lot about Cody's message, trying to figure it out. I got nowhere. That's no surprise because our brains evolved to make connections among things of *this* world. Cody was clearly communicating from somewhere else. So I couldn't solve the riddle by thinking.

I had a lot of feelings too. I was touched that Cody was concerned enough to send me that message. He was always sweet and considerate. One time he gave me a birthday card and wrote inside that I should only reply to his good wishes if it was convenient for me. I couldn't remember anyone else being that thoughtful. But feelings didn't solve the riddle either.

That central LSD question came up too. If *you* are always the same *you* regardless of whether you have an ego or even a self—who was Cody when he sent me that message?

Could the real *you* persist after you die?

Cody continued on to wherever people go after they die, and to the best of my knowledge, he didn't return. Yet somehow he found a way to let me know he was fine.

Finally I gave up on both thinking and feeling. I ended up just wondering. It was a mystery. I remembered a quote from Albert Einstein. He said that wondering and mystery were the source of all great art and science, and that anyone who couldn't stand in wonder, wrapped in awe, was as good as dead.

> Could the real you persist after you die?

That was it. The word that most closely describes how I experienced the message from Cody was *awe*. It reminded me of how I felt as a teenager when my girlfriend and I sat outside at night and looked up at the stars. The universe felt immeasurably immense, like a huge abyss, and we felt so small. That made me feel wonderful, for what reason I couldn't imagine. I just wasn't mature enough to recognize awe.

I began to appreciate awe. I cultivated it. When I moved to the San Francisco Bay area, I took notice of how I felt the first time I stood quietly in a virgin redwood forest. Having been raised in the woods of Pennsylvania, I was always comfortable among the trees.

But those ancient giants affected me like no other forest ever had. They stopped my mind.

When you're awestruck, they say you're *struck dumb*. Yes, when you're awestruck, you're slack-jawed and you can't say a word. More importantly, when you're awestruck, that incessant voice in your head finally shuts up.

Once my mind was out of the way, I could hear the redwoods. They were speaking to me without words. *We've been waiting for you*, they said.

I nodded inside, registering that I'd heard. So they continued.

We have things to teach. But nobody seems to listen.

I just closed my eyes and breathed. The quietness was sacred.

The redwoods taught me, and I learned an important lesson. Once my mind was quiet, I knew who I was.

CHAPTER 3

Camp Wheeze

"What did you do to those kids?"

The Professor glared at me from behind his desk. He was angry, which was hard to understand. I had organized a research project to benefit kids with severe asthma, and the results had been surprisingly good.

Admittedly, my methods were a little unorthodox. The Professor was a well-respected clinician and researcher. When it came to medical interventions, he went by the book.

The problem was, I was no longer willing to do that. I was approaching the end of my third year of medical school. It was summertime, but I couldn't take time off.

After Mr. Crawford died, I saw many other patients with rare diseases, and all of them were seriously ill. They were all treated the same way as Mr. Crawford. The standard medical approach to serious illness seemed clear: attack the disease with the most potent weapons available. Then, once the battle was over, survey the battlefield—the patient's body and psyche—and check to see if everything was okay.

In cases where the patient wasn't cured—which was almost all cases, as the diseases in question were chronic and incurable—the patient was most definitely not okay.

Many of these patients died. Their families went home empty-handed—not only without their loved ones, but also without any more understanding, confidence, or comfort than they'd brought with them when they arrived. These cases all reinforced my Learning Experience with Mr. Crawford.

They taught me that I needed to find another source of learning. It seemed obvious to me that in our attempts to cure, we had forgotten about healing. In fact, healing never came up. But I wanted to learn about healing as much as I wanted to learn about curing. So I decided to graduate early.

The lesson from the redwoods was also fresh in my mind. When my mind stopped, I knew who I was. Unfortunately, stopping your mind is impossible while you're on duty in an academic medical center. It follows that many people in that setting are not familiar with who they really are, at least while they're at work.

I thought that learning how to be a healer might be associated with learning who you really are—and with the learning that resulted from stopping your mind.

So I learned to meditate. It's the handiest and most effective way to stop your mind—and after a while, sure enough, you get more familiar with who you really are. When I say *after a while*, bear in mind that all this happened fifty years ago. You can't rush these things.

To earn enough credits to graduate early, I needed to work through the summer. Since there were no clerkships in the summer, I had to get creative.

Learning about meditation made me curious about guided imagery and visualization. Was it possible to influence the body through proper use of the mind? Even better, might using the mind in the right way help remedy illness?

If there was one illness that visualization could help, I thought it might be asthma. People with severe asthma have highly reactive airways. They tighten up in reaction to many allergens—springtime pollen and wintertime mold spores are the most common.

But asthmatic patients' airways also tighten during times of stress and emotional tension. What would happen, I wondered, if there were a way to help these patients relax emotionally? Would their airways relax too?

I designed a simple pilot study, typed it up, and took it over to the university children's hospital. They had a whole wing devoted to childhood asthma. These kids had asthma attacks that were frequent and severe. Their parents were constantly on high alert. The moment the wheezing started, the parents would throw their child into the car and streak to the emergency room. Often the child flew right through the ER and ended up in the pediatric ICU. In the most severe cases, the child's airways were so tight, and responded so poorly to treatment, that the child would progress to respiratory failure and even death.

When I arrived to meet the Professor, he had already formed an opinion about my project. "So you believe you can hypnotize these kids and cure their asthma?" he asked.

I explained that visualization is different from hypnosis. I'd teach them to sit down, close their eyes, breathe slow and easy, and see a movie in their head. I would meet with them once a week for six weeks and teach them a different visualization exercise each time. They would practice at home. We'd keep track of how many asthma attacks they had during the study and compare those numbers with their usual attack rate.

He frowned, then had to admit that he couldn't see any risk to the kids. He approved the study, then picked ten kids who frequented the hospital and gave me permission to call their parents. When I contacted them, they were willing to try anything. All agreed to bring their kids in on the appointed day.

One of the social work students heard what I was doing and volunteered to assist. We had no budget, so we used our own money to buy white T-shirts, ten kid-size and two adults. Then we tie-dyed them red, orange, and yellow and stenciled CAMP WHEEZE on the front of each one in big black capital letters.

We were in business.

I standardized my preparation routine. I'd go to the hospital an hour before each meeting, find a quiet room, and sit down by myself. I'd meditate for a while and send out a mental request for a visualization. A nice one, different each time, would show up in my mind.

When the kids arrived, happily wearing their new T-shirts, we set up chairs in a circle outside on the lawn. The summer weather was invariably gorgeous—warm sun, no clouds or wind.

They were a great group. There was Juan, a skinny twelve-year-old with braces and a huge smile. Kerri was ten with pink glasses and a long brown ponytail. Then there was Kurt—six years old, blond and bouncy, with the sunniest disposition you could imagine. The other seven were just as appealing. All of them seemed excited and ready to explore.

We talked for a short while. Then I asked them to close their eyes and breathe easy. I invited them to come along on a little trip, then I walked them through the visualization. We went through this same routine each time we met.

One time, we hiked through a forest. Another time, we climbed a mountain until we got to the top where we could see for miles and the air was clear and pure. They loved that one. One day we went to the beach and walked into gentle waves, then just kept on walking. We found we could breathe underwater. Unfortunately, that one didn't go so well. Asthma and underwater breathing weren't very compatible. But we popped up to the surface and everyone was okay. At least nobody wound up in the hospital.

Four weeks into the study, the Professor called me into his office. "You've got some explaining to do," he said. "One of the parents called me. She demanded to know what you're doing with her son."

"What happened?" I asked. "Everything seems to be going well."

"She told me little Kurt started to wheeze. She was about to run him to the ER, but he told her to wait. He sat down on the couch and closed his eyes. His asthma went away."

Wow! Maybe this actually works. Maybe they'll want to study it.

No such luck. The Professor was not pleased. "I need you to tell me exactly what you're doing to those kids," he said.

"Wait," I said. "We went over the proposal in detail. I'm doing exactly what I described in there."

The professor looked incredulous. "You mean you're just telling those kids to close their eyes and see pictures?"

"Exactly," I said. "And we should consider the possibility that doing that has an effect on their physiology—and their psychology—that helps them deal with their asthma."

He looked up at the ceiling for several seconds. Then he looked back at me. "You're not doing a damn thing for those kids."

Wait! What about what Kurt's mother said?

He spat out his final conclusion in disgust. "You're just giving them love!"

The meeting was over. So was the project. I considered publishing a paper about it, but I knew it would be fruitless. We had a single interesting result, but no real data. Kurt's experience was just an anecdote. No journal would publish that.

And it was 1976. Even if I accumulated a whole list of events like Kurt's, all the editors of major peer-reviewed medical journals would harbor the same attitude as the Professor had—skeptical at best. I didn't want to imagine the worst.

Oh well. Another Learning Experience.

For the next several weeks, I performed my routine medical student duties at the hospital. At least I would get credit for the clerkship. During my last week, I was eating lunch in the cafeteria when the Head of Child Psychiatry pulled up a chair.

"Hey, word is getting around about your project," he said. "Our department agrees that guided visualization may have potential in asthma. Are you interested in making your little intervention operational?"

"I'm not sure," I said. "It doesn't seem to be getting a good reception."

"On the contrary," he said. "We think you may be onto something. I can't make any concrete offers yet, but would you consider helping us start a clinic for asthmatic kids here? We'd be doing both therapeutics and research."

I perked my ears up at that. It would be refreshing to work on some new ideas and actually get support for them. I told him I'd give it some thought, and we could meet again in a week. I would just be finishing my summer clerkship then, and I'd be getting ready to graduate.

We never had that second meeting. The Professor objected to the clinic and refused to let any of his patients participate.

Just a few of us graduated in September. There was no cap and gown, no going up on stage to receive my diploma, no pomp and circumstance.

Only Learning Experiences.

When the Professor told me I hadn't done anything for those kids, I didn't take it personally. He was simply biased. In a way, that didn't fit because researchers like him are trained to eliminate bias. But scientists are always biased in favor of established, proven beliefs. It takes more convincing to change their minds than just anecdotal evidence from one little Kurt. So I wasn't surprised that he rejected the message that Kurt's mother had delivered.

But, when he told me that the *nothing* I'd given those kids was *just love*, I had to draw the line.

Love means nothing? Come on. No human being, at least one dedicated to healing, could let that statement go.

It was time to find some new teachers. Lucky for me, there turned out to be plenty of really good ones.

My patients.

CHAPTER 4

Love on the Leukemia Ward

As I poked my head into his room, Chas swiveled his head on the pillow and gave me a gap-tooth grin.

"So Chas," I asked, pulling a chair up next to his bed, "how did you lose your left front tooth?"

"The sonofabitch in the bar was right-handed."

Chas was a Hell's Angel. Over years of riding the San Jose freeways, flying gravel had chipped some of his other teeth. As the dentist's office was not his favorite place, several of his teeth were blackened. This was a red flag. Bacteria thriving in rotten teeth can wreak havoc on patients who are receiving chemotherapy for acute leukemia.

By this time, I was an intern in 1978. Chas was my patient—truly mine. His oncologist, my attending, turned him over to me after Chas was readmitted with a 104 degree fever, chills, and cough just two weeks after his initial chemotherapy. Dr. Clark, a stoop-shouldered, white-haired physician nearing retirement, had long since burned out from exposure to decades of treatment failure, tragedy, and death.

"You take him," he said, slumped in a chair behind his desk. "I can't stand watching one more young person die. You make the decisions, everything but the chemo. Come to me about that. But don't call about anything else unless you run into problems you can't handle yourself."

What a gift, I thought. *Just a year out of medical school, and I can make my own decisions.*

I was comfortable taking over Chas's case, except for one little detail. I wasn't comfortable with Chas. He and all his buddies were complete aliens to me. Every time I laid eyes on them, I had to brace myself for a new wave of culture shock. Talk about a barrier to the doctor-patient relationship.

I had a lot of judgments about Chas. They were embarrassing even to me. I saw him as a low-life slacker, maybe a lawbreaker, probably a liar. I wasn't sure I could believe a word he told me.

Chas was twenty-four, about my age, but the resemblance ended there. I was a middle-class guy, training day and night for an elite profession. He was a part-time garage mechanic who didn't give a damn whether his job would still be there when (or if) he got out of the hospital.

In fact, he didn't give a rip about anything but his motorcycle. He talked about it all the time. He kept a framed 8 × 10 photo of it on his bedside table. "I cherried that baby out," he said. "Three coats of red metal-flake paint topped with five coats of clear lacquer."

As for me, I hated motorcycles. Some people may get excited seeing the pavement whiz by underneath at 90 mph, with nothing but air between them and their destiny. I was not one of those people.

In the ER, I'd seen bikers brought in dead after crashes, flesh scraped off their bones by the asphalt, necks fractured, brains reduced to mush extruding through cracks in their shorty helmets. Depending on the specifics of the case, we would call those big Harley hogs either *suicycles* or *murdercycles*.

Chas and I had other personal differences. For instance, most days I'd take a shower. If he hadn't been enjoying the bed baths the nurses gave him, Chas wouldn't have bothered to clean up. His friends certainly didn't. Shaggy groups of brother Angels hung out in Chas's room every day, clad in T-shirts with the sleeves ripped off. Although those shirts must have started out white, they had long since devolved to a greasy yellowish-gray. Over the T-shirts, they wore faded, ripped denim vests smeared with grease and road dirt. On the back, the Hells Angels' name glowed in bright red block letters on a white background arched over a golden flying death's head—a laughing skull in profile trailing a glorious array of red and gold flames like the intermingling of a raptor's wings, a tribal chieftain's royal headdress, and a helmet on fire.

I regretted my attitude, but I had no one to discuss it with. My burned-out attending oncologist was clearly not the person to consult, and it would be years before anyone would provide support groups and counseling for interns and residents. This was my baggage, and I had to carry it.

All day, Chas and his buddies sat, ignoring his shaky situation, laughing and scratching like they were sharing the biggest joke in the world. When visiting hours were over, the Angels filed out his door cackling wildly, their laughter echoing up and down the hall. Once the elevator doors slid shut behind them, the nurses followed with spray cans.

Chas's biker friends were imposing specimens. Bo was nearly seven feet tall with a gold stud in his left earlobe and snakes tattooed up and down both arms. He had to bend over to fit through the door to the hospital room. Steve was a short stubby guy with a long black beard. His butt was so wide his haunches must have lapped over the sides of his seat like saddlebags. His jeans hung low, his beer belly protruding out from under his T-shirt. After he finally shoehorned himself into one of the hospital chairs, he swayed back and forth, rubbing his belly with both hands like a Santa Claus from hell. Occasionally he'd boost himself to his feet and bend over the bedrail, butt crack exposed, offering a glass of water to Chas with surprising tenderness.

As I watched, I was forced to admit the Angels were a close-knit bunch of losers.

Chas might have bulked up in the past, but cancer had made him so frail and wispy that it seemed opening the window might blow him out of bed. He had acute myelogenous leukemia, or AML. This cancer results when a clone of leukocytes, the white blood cells that fight bacterial infections, go rogue and multiply wildly, crowding normal blood-forming cells out of the bone marrow. The clinical picture was similar to Mr. Crawford's—it just involved a different kind of white blood cell.

AML progresses rapidly. Chas's type is invariably fatal weeks to months after diagnosis unless it is treated with aggressive chemotherapy. Even then, long-term survival is rare.

AML transforms the genes of leukocytes at an early stage of their development. The worst types of AML involve genetic mutations in white blood cells while they are still *blasts*, so immature that they are basically infants, unable to perform any of the adult functions of leukocytes.

Blasts flood out of the marrow into the bloodstream. Soon vast numbers of them swarm throughout the circulation, all stuck at the same stage of immaturity. It's like a horror movie where hordes of babies take over the city.

Since blasts can't perform any of the functions of adult white cells, they're incapable of attacking and ingesting bacteria like adult leukocytes do. In short order, patients with AML fall prey to bacterial infections of all kinds. The final common pathway of any unchecked bacterial infection is *septicemia* or blood poisoning, which is rapidly and uniformly fatal unless it's treated with intravenous antibiotics.

But antibiotics alone can't cure septicemia. Antibiotic therapy requires an intact immune system, particularly a healthy crop of leukocytes, to be effective. Because the marrow is packed with blasts, functional leukocytes are in short supply. AML inflicts a double whammy on its patients: they are infected easily, and it's hard for them to fight infections once they start.

Chas had already failed his first round of chemo. AML patients initially undergo *induction* chemotherapy, consisting of several drugs given in large doses over just a few days. As happened with Mr. Crawford, this amounts to an all-out assault on the leukemia cells in the bone marrow. Most or all of those malignant cells succumb, along with a large proportion of the healthy blood-forming cells.

If all goes well, the healthy cells take off and repopulate the marrow, renewing the supply of white cells, red cells, and platelets in the bloodstream. Any remaining leukemia cells are then controlled with *consolidation* chemotherapy, employing a different cocktail of less toxic drugs that selectively destroy them while leaving healthy marrow cells relatively unscathed. That's the theory, anyway.

AML recurs in most cases because the leukemia cells develop resistance to chemotherapy drugs, like bacteria do to antibiotics. Thus AML is rarely curable, except for a few unusual subtypes. I've seen patients who were cured—they dodged death, but its shadow continued to cloud their horizons. In usual cases of AML, chemotherapy can buy scant periods of time for patients who do respond.

Unlike Mr. Crawford, Chas had responded to his original induction. His blast levels declined significantly, although not to zero. Still, he almost died in the process. The healthy leukocytes in his bloodstream vanished, and pneumonia and sepsis put him in the ICU for a week. He made it out to the ward, then to discharge. After he got home, he felt better at first, but soon the dreaded fatigue and loss of appetite returned, then fever and cough. Leukemia cells again flooded his circulation.

Chas hadn't made it to consolidation chemo. He was now admitted for IV antibiotics, then reinduction. His ordeal was about to start all over again.

There had to be a way to connect with him. As a doctor, I would need to learn to work with patients I didn't like. If I could find a way to do that, I might be able to discover what Chas really wanted. That way our medical juggernaut might not run right over him.

The first two days of this current admission had been taken up with tests and procedures, with no time for small talk. I came in for rounds the third morning.

"Hey Doc," said Chas. "What am I in for this time?"

"It's called reinduction chemotherapy," I replied. "It's pretty much a replay of what you went through the first time around."

This did not reassure him. "Whoa man, seriously? You guys just about killed me."

"This chemo is a big deal," I said. "No point in denying it. It's rough, but it has to be if you want to handle the leukemia." *Not* your *leukemia*, I thought. *It might be good to put some distance between Chas and the disease.*

"Why in hell would I ever want to go through that again?" he asked.

Deep breath. Time for truth. "Because leukemia is fatal if you don't treat it," I said.

"Fatal? You mean I'm going to die?

"It's hard to say. Treatment may knock it back." I was lying. We planned to use the same drug combination that had failed the first time.

"Haha! You're saying *may*, not *will*. Come on, level with me, Doc."

I sighed. "Okay, it's *may* because there's no guarantee it will work."

"It sure didn't the first time."

"Actually it did, sort of." I couldn't resist grabbing onto a slim strand of hope. *Is that hope for him or for me?* "The chemo pretty much took care of the leukemia," I said. "You got out of the hospital, and things went back to normal. For a while."

"Right," he sneered. "For how long? I went through hell, and now I'm back here. Less than a month. Doesn't sound like it worked to me."

I sighed again. "I hear you," I said. "No guarantee things will be much different this time."

Silence.

Chas considered what I'd just said. "What would you do?" he asked. "If it was your life?"

That was a fair question. "I'd have to think about it for a while," I said. "I'd probably say to myself: 'What would you give up for a little more life? Is it worth going all out, all over again?'"

I remembered Mr. Crawford. It had seemed so natural to imagine not treating him. Now I found myself on the other side of the question. "I don't know what my answer would be," I said. "But I'm not the one who's up against it here."

Now it was Chas's turn to sigh. "Yeah. That would be me."

"I guess you've got some thinking to do," I said. "You're the one on the hot seat. I'll be back tomorrow, and we'll see what we can come up with."

"Sounds good," he said.

We looked at each other. Something had just happened between us.

We are in this together.

I walked in the next morning to find a young woman standing by Chas's bed. The two of them were engaged in earnest conversation. She was tall, nearly six feet, thin and statuesque, wearing tight black pants and a beige top that was even tighter. She was striking, but her most arresting feature was the dyed blond Afro that crowned her head. It must have measured a foot and a half across. It was impeccably maintained.

"Hi," she said. "I'm Felice, Chas's girlfriend."

I tried to make small talk, but she got right to the point. "Chas says this chemo isn't going to do anything but make him miserable."

By this time, I had relinquished my sense of duty to treatment. But I still felt compelled to present both sides. "We don't know that," I said. "It may buy him time."

"Come on Doc, cut the crap," she snapped. "You and I both know he's going to die."

Well now. That's one point we won't have to haggle over. "Okay, yeah," I said.

"So Chas and I have been talking," she went on. "If he doesn't have much time left, we want to get married."

The conversation was now moving so fast that I had trouble keeping up. "Uh, I'm not sure how to pull that off," I stammered.

"I know a priest," she said. "Let's get him in here."

I hesitated, mind racing, then surrendered. "Well . . . why not?" *Hey, they told me I could make the decisions.*

In these situations, it's important to be strategic. So I got the nurses involved. In any hospital, once they get behind a plan, the outcome is inevitable. Most of them thought the marriage was a great idea, even the Charge Nurse. It didn't hurt that they'd gotten to know Bo and Steve, who were charming on a good day. The hospital administration gave their blessing. A Hells Angels' wedding on the cancer ward would be great for community relations.

Chas was fading, so the big day arrived almost immediately. Chas, Felice, Bo, Steve, and a couple of other Angels crammed into Chas's room along with the priest. He was as depraved as everyone else, dressed in black tie and tails with a tight braid halfway down his back and a knife through a heart tattooed up his neck.

They closed the door. Before long, pot smoke wafted out from underneath, along with lots of shrieking and clapping.

Before long, the party broke up and the door flew open. Bo banged his head against the doorframe on the way out. Chas's buddies stumbled off, smoke drifting down the hall after them.

Chas sprawled in bed with a blissful smile on his face as Felice reclined in a chair by the bedside.

I said, "Nice job, you two."

"You too," they replied in unison. We all giggled.

The next morning I came in for rounds. Chas was propped up on pillows, gazing at a glossy magazine. "Hey Doc, c'mere," he said. "You gotta check this out."

I sat down on the bed by Chas's side and gazed at a motorcycle magazine, the double centerfold spread wide open on his lap. There in magnificent splendor shined a gorgeous candy-apple red Harley Davidson, chrome sparkling. The editors of the biker magazine had heard about Chas. His story went national. Now every biker in the country could behold his pride and joy.

Then I did a doubletake. Draped across the handlebars was a voluptuous, totally nude young woman—with a huge blond Afro.

"Ain't she beautiful?" crowed Chas.

I had no idea if he was referring to his bike, or his new wife, or both. And it didn't matter. They were both gorgeous.

Chas decided against any more chemo. We arranged for him to be discharged to Felice's apartment. I broke free from the hospital to visit them a couple of times. He slept in a hospital bed in the living room for a week and a half until he died, peacefully and without pain.

Chas and Felice were both happy to see me when I showed up. The feeling was mutual. That just goes to show you: healing goes both ways.

The same year I met Chas and Felice, an article titled "Taking Care of the Hateful Patient" appeared in the New England Journal of Medicine (Groves 1978). The author described four types of patients that doctors hate: dependent clingers, entitled demanders, manipulative help-rejecters, and self-destructive deniers.

Many physicians read and commented on that article, but nobody made the obvious comment: it missed the point.

Labeling patients as dependent, entitled, demanding, or self-destructive takes the doctor off the hook. The burden is not on the patient to be free of psychological issues or personality disorders. The burden is on the doctor to let go of judgments and to *be* in the room—to get on the same side of the table as the person with the problems.

At our first meeting, I didn't dislike Chas because he had psychological issues. I disliked him because he was different from me, radically different. In fact, he was that way on purpose. Hell's Angels don't act, dress, or smell the way they do in order to conform to other people's expectations.

> The burden is on the doctor to let go of judgments and to be in the room— to get on the same side of the table as the person with the problems.

If I was going to get to the bottom of Chas's challenges and be of any real help to him as a person, not just as the owner of a disease I couldn't cure—it was up to me to get past all the stuff in the way. Nine times out of ten, that stuff is mine.

This is a choice all healers must make. Why? Because healing requires you to get as close as you can to another person who is suffering, without drifting away from your own center and merging with their challenges. Once you cross that line, you're no longer helpful.

But as a healer, there's another line that you must cross: your own fear. Not fear of death—everybody has that.

The line a healer must cross: Fear of your own feelings.

Emotional Resonance

Getting close to another person who's suffering is guaranteed to ring your own bells. When another person is in anguish and you allow yourself to get close enough to help, that closeness will inevitably engage your own feelings.

This is an occupational risk for physicians. It's related to empathy, but it's not the same. Empathy allows you to feel what another person is feeling. Empathy is vital in healing.

> ## The line a healer must cross: Fear of your own feelings.

Emotional resonance is more like sympathy. You don't just feel; you react unconsciously as your own bells get rung. If you don't notice that your own chimes are ringing, one of two things will happen: Either you'll suffer right along with that person, or you'll check out. Either way, you've been pulled out of your own center, whether you realize it or not.

At that point, you're useless.

Healing Your Self

Emotional resonance happens to everyone—at first. If you want to be a healer, you experience it, then notice it. Then, a critical step: you learn to hold back judgments against yourself for feeling it. You have to learn to forgive your self. After all, you can't blame your self. Its purpose is just to learn.

The next and most crucial step is to *feel* those emotions fully. That's mindfulness. Only after you feel them fully can you let them go.

You may notice that when you're being truly mindful, you're occupying a particular place inside your own consciousness. It's the place where *you* live. You're just aware. No thoughts. Your mind has stopped. You're bringing your emotions to that place, and it's easy to do because the place itself is empty.

As you enter that emptiness, that place where you are nothing but aware, that's when you become who you really are. When you first experience

46

this, you may not even notice it. This fundamental element of your awareness is subtle, but crucial.

Learning to inhabit this place is what the practice of healing is all about. Only when you *are* in that place of pure awareness can you truly *be*. And only then can you truly *be with* another human being.

Truly being with someone who's suffering can transform them. It can set them on the road toward healing. But it also transforms the healer because it reveals the difference between being truly aware and simply being aware of their self.

The place of true *being* is the only place in this world that's perfect. That's a new slant on *practice makes perfect*.

The Hand-on-the-Doorknob Syndrome

Too many people—including many doctors—avoid situations that require them to get close to suffering. Others may get close physically, pretending to listen to the anguish of people struggling to cope with the news that they can't be cured. These pretenders may appear to listen, but they don't really hear.

I refer to this as *The Hand-on-the-Doorknob Syndrome*. Someday, a doctor afflicted with this condition may be sitting right in front of you as you speak about your suffering. He may appear to be listening. But if you look carefully, you will see that he really wants to be out in the hallway. He wants to apply the classic physician coping maneuver: moving on to the next case.

Many patients and their loved ones sense this, so they don't bring up their feelings to the doctor at all. It's not just that they know they won't be heard. Also, they don't want to upset the doctor. It's an instance of power inequality, like when children avoid saying things they know will upset their parents.

Parents have the advantage of time. They may learn to listen as their children grow, eventually becoming teenagers who have no trouble saying whatever is on their minds. But physicians don't have that long to wait. Their frightened patients may not have time to grow. You can't suddenly become mature when you're suffering and afraid. More commonly, people regress when their life is threatened.

Deep Listening

It's the doctor's responsibility to sit face to face with a patient, ask the right questions, and then listen—deeply.

Unfortunately, most doctors today aren't face to face with anyone. They're looking at their keyboards as they type data into the medical record. Some doctors have assistants enter the data so the doctor can face the patient. But transcribers cost money, so most practices don't employ them.

If you want to engage in healing, you need to listen differently. Healers sit down eye to eye with people who are suffering, take a deep breath, and open their ears, hearts, and minds to hear what that person is really talking about.

> Learn to center your self in the real you.

To become a healer, you need to start by knowing who you really are. Learn to center your self in the real *you*. Once you do, you never know what's going to happen. But transformation may be on the table—for everyone involved.

CHAPTER 5

Man Down

It was 2:00 a.m. on a winter night. Two inches of fresh snow covered the ground, so the ER wasn't busy.

Like many rural ERs, this one was staffed with a close-knit clinical team. Lucia, the nurse, was gruff but gentle. She lived in a converted railroad caboose and wore cowboy boots under her purple scrubs. She was a professional in all the best ways. She knew how to stay calm in a crisis. She would talk down crazy guys with guns—and she had plenty of opportunities. There were a lot of meth labs in the county. Best of all, Lucia knew how to laugh.

I'll never forget how she oriented me on my first day. "Here's the prime rule, Dr. Stuart," she said. "Sexual harassment will not be reported. But it will be graded."

Carl the LVN was a tall, quiet guy with enough muscle to back up Lucia if needed. Lou was the guard with the badge. He never carried a gun because he didn't need one. He was built like a side of beef and weighed about the same.

Kitty was the receptionist. She also monitored the radio. Like everyone else, she knew how to keep her cool. One night her dad, who had terrible lung disease, came in unconscious in respiratory failure, lips and fingers blue. I told her we had thirty seconds to decide before I would be forced to put a tube down his windpipe and place him on a ventilator. He'd been on the vent in the ICU before and hated every second of it. So Kitty decided to let her dad go. We rolled his gurney into a back room where it was quiet and gave him morphine until he was comfortable. He died within an hour. Kitty checked him periodically and kissed him goodbye. But she always kept one ear tuned to the radio.

One snowy night when I was on duty, a young mom put her three-year-old son into his car seat and didn't bother to belt him in. Visibility was poor. She pulled out of the driveway into the path of an oncoming truck. Two separate ambulances brought them in. The little boy had an obvious skull fracture and was already gone. The mom had sustained a concussion but was still semi-conscious.

I spent a couple of hours removing glass fragments and repairing multiple lacerations of her face. When I was almost done, I felt a tap on my shoulder. It was one of the local deputy sheriffs. We knew each other well. "Oh, hi Ron," I said.

"Sorry to poke my head in, Doc," he replied. "But when your patient wakes up, I have some business to do."

"Yeah," I said. "Very unfortunate about the seatbelt."

In this world, misfortune can build fast. You could feel it happening that night. As the surgical and police work proceeded, Lucia called the father and told him to come right down. He arrived just as his wife was waking up. I brought him into the room where she lay on the gurney, still somewhat dazed but able to comprehend what I needed to tell them. I offered him a chair beside his wife.

The father asked about their son. I said that some terrible things had happened. The mother gasped and put her hand to her mouth. I asked if the two of them were okay with my telling them the details. Looking warily at each other, they agreed.

I told them their son had been badly injured, so badly he couldn't recover. And that the deputy sheriff was waiting to take the mother to jail.

It was good that the mother was lying on the gurney with the bed rails up. The father was not so fortunate. He fell out of his chair onto the floor, screaming and writhing on the linoleum like he was possessed. Which he was—by overwhelming shock and horror.

I knelt beside him and put my hand on his shoulder. Slowly his convulsions slowed until he was just wrenched by wracking sobs.

> At times, the act of healing may be limited to a simple comforting hand.

Some events are so truly unspeakable that words are out of place. At times, the act of healing may be limited to a simple comforting hand.

That night Kitty called out, "Man down in the shower unconscious, V-tach, rate 240, BP 50 over undetectable. ETA four minutes."

Translated into English, that means a man was found collapsed in his shower. Ventricular tachycardia had elevated his heart rate so high he couldn't generate sufficient blood pressure to sustain brain function and consciousness.

The doors blew open and snow flew in. The EMTs ran the gurney to the treatment room and tore the man's shirt open to expose his bare chest. I had the paddles ready and immediately shocked him.

Today, California regulations would allow the EMTs to shock the patient as soon as they arrived at his house and again enroute. But that was not legal practice in 1991. That night his heart stayed in its non-functional rhythm for an extra fifteen minutes.

The first electroshock did nothing. The patient stayed in V-tach. We all pitched in to throw the patient from the gurney onto the treatment table. He was a very large man.

Only when we had him positioned did Lucia get a chance to look at his face.

"Good Christ, it's Lou!" she screamed. She had tears in her eyes. I had never seen her get emotional.

This resuscitation was now personal. That wouldn't alter anything we would do, but the tone in the room had changed. In the blink of an eye, the atmosphere flashed from calmly professional to desperately grim.

We tried everything. Nothing worked. Lou's V-tach degenerated into ventricular fibrillation, then asystole—flat line.

Lou probably had a clot in a major coronary artery—the primary cause of heart attacks—blocking blood flow to a large portion of his heart muscle, starving it of oxygen and causing electrical instability and lethal rhythm problems. The only remedy would have been cardiac catheterization and stenting or coronary bypass surgery. But the nearest cath lab was an hour away by helicopter. Before we could load him up and fly him out, we needed to resuscitate Lou and stabilize him.

There was no point in calling the helicopter.

I've always hated TV medical dramas. On TV, patients survive cardiac arrest and resuscitation as if it were just a bad cold, only shorter in duration. In real life, most people who suffer cardiac arrest end up like Lou.

After thirty minutes of fruitless CPR, I decided we were done. "I'm calling the code," I said.

No one disagreed. We had lost the fight. And we'd lost a friend. Everyone backed away from the table, heads hanging, defeated.

A failed code is always a dismal scene. This one was abysmal.

I headed to the phone to dictate a note. When I came back, the mortuary staff was loading Lou's body into the hearse. Lucia wasn't around. That was strange. Normally she would be busy running everything.

I found her in the back, leaning face first against the wall. Her shoulders were shaking. I put my hand on her back. She nodded. That was it. Once again, a healing hand took the place of empty words.

The ER can be a choke point for tragedy. That was one of those nights. Sudden death is merciless. There's no time to prepare. One terrible moment yanks lives apart.

Chronic illness is different. When you're diagnosed, that's your yellow light. You'd better beware—and prepare. But sudden death is a red light. Everything stops. The damage is done and there's no return. It's irreparable. No one gets to adjust.

All the survivors can do is pick up the pieces. That night, the survivors were us. The pieces were inside, where no one could see.

Kitty announced another ambulance was arriving. We grabbed a breath and moved on.

Sudden death is impossible for the rational mind to handle. It's almost intolerable—but not quite.

If you witness enough deaths, you will begin to notice a pattern. All the deaths you see will have one factor in common. You won't notice it at first. Only later will it dawn on you.

You didn't die. It's always somebody else.

In the ultimate sense, death doesn't exist. That center of your awareness where you really reside, the real *you*, arrived as you were born, and that real *you* moves on when the body dies.

But in a very earthly sense, death doesn't exist for your regular, earthly self either. Because it always happens to somebody else. Your regular self will never experience death.

That's because when you die, your regular self dies too. Once you're dead, there's no self there to experience it.

Woody Allen said, "I'm not afraid of death. I just don't want to be there when it happens."

Well, you won't be.

All this talk about the real *you* and your ordinary self may sound like empty words or philosophic mumbo jumbo. But it's not. It's the difference between this world and the eternal.

None of this occurred to me until I'd witnessed many deaths. One day, it dawned on me that the real *me*—the Witness within me—is the only part of me that actually understands death. Only that central place in my consciousness really grasps its meaning. That real *me* takes in the experience of this moment, then goes on to the next moment, and then the next. Like beads on a string. It's like the quantum theory of life.

One moment, that person is over there. The next moment they're not. To your earthly self, those moments seem so unbearably different. But to the real *you*, it's all the same.

After you've been through enough loss, you will gain some depth perspective.

Once that happens, you can start to see the difference between *loss*— which is integral to life in this world, which the real *you* understands—and *grief*, your ordinary self's reaction to loss.

This is not to minimize grief. Many people tell me, and I have experienced it myself, that when you lose someone important, you never really recover. A hole with the shape of that person lives on within you. Grief can be devastating at first and debilitating for much longer. Many other authors have approached grief with grace and elegance I can't match.

If you want to learn about healing, however, you have to learn the difference between the real *you* and your ordinary self. They are both real— from the perspective of this world. But from the perspective of the eternal, your ordinary self is only real for a time—and time does not exist. Only the real *you* is eternally real.

> Only the real you is eternally real.

Don't let your mind convince you that believing this will solve your problem with death. It won't because no belief will. It's just the first step on the journey toward finding out who you really are.

That won't totally solve your problem either. But it will get you well on the way.

CHAPTER 6

Lightning Rounds

Mrs. Dinucci slumped fast asleep in a wheelchair beside her hospital bed. She was seventy-six, haggard and scrawny, clad only in a purple fuzzy robe, her mottled ankles sticking out the bottom. Her dry, cracked heels, only partly covered by hospital-issue green paper slippers, rested on the linoleum. Wisps of brown hair streaked with silver straggled over her forehead. Ravaged by lung cancer, radiation, and two rounds of chemotherapy, she was admitted for yet another session of chemo the next morning.

I was in my first year of practice, on weekend call for my group. If it hadn't been for my four call partners, I would have been on call 24 hours a day, 7 days a week, 365 days a year. But the tradeoff was that I had to see every patient that each of my partners and I had admitted to the hospital and take phone calls from all my partners' practices, the hospitals, and the Emergency Room. It wasn't unusual to field hundreds of calls from 5 p.m. Friday until 9 a.m. Monday.

On that Sunday morning, I had twenty-four patients to see for five different doctors in three different hospitals. I was making *lightning rounds.* I started early in the morning, and I knew I had to move fast to have any chance of seeing my kids before they were in bed. And I wanted to get a little sleep myself among all the phone calls and runs to the ER that would happen all night, before I had to be back in the hospital at sunrise on Monday morning.

Mrs. Dinucci was my partner's patient. I had never met her before. I was tempted just to glance at her, make sure she was tuned up and ready for chemo, and move on. The oncologist would be seeing her in an hour or two anyway.

But something made me linger. I watched her bony chest rise and fall as she snored quietly. I thought of other patients I'd known with advanced non-small cell lung cancer. They waited with breathless expectation for treatment they hoped would slow the inexorable march of their disease. Instead, it often brought them pain, nausea, and vomiting throughout the scant few weeks or months they had left.

Mrs. Dinucci's hands were folded in her lap. Her red nail polish was chipped. Her red lipstick almost matched, even though breakfast had smeared it. The bony joint where her collarbone met the top of her shoulder blade poked out from inside her robe. I touched it gently.

She woke up and registered the stethoscope hanging around my neck. Her bloodshot, yellowed eyes opened wide and filled with tears. Her pale, parched lips, turned down at the corners, started to quiver.

So much for lightning rounds. I introduced myself and asked how she was doing. I didn't ask her what was wrong. I thought she should take the lead.

She got right to the point. "Doctor! I don't want this treatment," she said.

I must have looked puzzled.

"I'm serious!" she exclaimed. "They told me the chemo didn't shrink my cancer."

"That's got to be hard for you," I said.

"It is," she replied. "But that's not the worst part. I know I'm dying. But nobody will talk about it!" A tear ran down her sunken cheek, streaking her makeup.

I thought back to Chas's case several years before. It had taken some time and some talking—and his girlfriend's support—before he decided to forego cancer treatment. But Mrs. Dinucci had already made up her mind.

I could feel her anguish. I wanted to help, but I wasn't sure how. Luckily, I had a straw to grab. Just the week before, as the idealistic new doctor in town, I'd been invited to join the hospital Ethics Committee. The doctrine of informed consent was just coming into general use. It stated that patients have the right to know all the important details they need to make good choices about their care—then they get to decide for themselves.

Obviously, I was the one to introduce this principal to the patient. I decide to adopt a mature physician's demeanor. "Well, you know, Mrs. Dinucci," I intoned, "a patient doesn't have to do just what the doctor wants. Your treatment is up to you. You have the right to decide."

She stopped sniffling and stared at me. "Hah!" she snorted. "You have no idea. It's my family that needs me to have this treatment! It's not up to me."

I knew what the next step ought to be: a family meeting. But this was my partner's patient, not mine. I felt like kicking myself. *This could take hours. I'll never get home!*

Then a conviction familiar to all doctors overrode my caution. *Maybe there's something here I can fix.* "Are any of your family here today?" I asked. "Maybe we could talk together."

A broad smile creased her wrinkled face. "Really? That would be wonderful!"

I poked my head out into the hall. It was packed with visitors. Knots of men in blue suits and women in staid wool dresses chatted in the same hushed, respectful tones they had no doubt just used in church. I had no trouble being heard. I called out, "Is anyone here from Mrs. Dinucci's family?"

Roughly half the visitors in the hall turned toward me. Within minutes, sixteen people had packed into the room. Some sat, some stood shoulder to shoulder, some leaned on the walls. The crowd included parents, brothers and sisters, spouses, and children. Two grandchildren sat on the bed, playing with little plastic farm animals. Once everyone was settled, they looked at me expectantly.

"Mrs. Dinucci and I have talked," I began. "There are a few things we'd like to discuss with you all. Mrs. Dinucci, would you like to start us off?"

The patient was now hunched down in her wheelchair as if her body had shrunk several sizes. Her chin barely protruded above the neck of her purple bathrobe. She stared straight ahead. Her face seemed made of stone except for her jaw muscles, which jerked in a helter-skelter rhythm. "No," she said with finality.

"Um, okay," I mumbled.

In the hushed room, every eye was fixed on my face. Finally, I blurted out the one solitary notion that bobbed, flashing like a harbor buoy, on the surface of my mind. "Mrs. Dinucchi is not sure she wants to go through with the chemotherapy scheduled for tomorrow," I said. "She doesn't think her treatment is helping. In fact, she recognizes that she's probably going to die." *There, the ice is broken.*

The silence that followed was ended by a grunt from an old but very large man sitting in a chair in the far corner of the room. He heaved himself upright and walked slowly toward me. The crowd parted to make room for him to pass. He cleaved through the sea of family members like a steamship. Dressed in overalls and a plaid flannel shirt, he was at least six foot four and proportionately wide.

He's aged well. And he's in shape.

As he reached the place where I stood, he brought the tips of his cracked tan work boots toe to toe with my wingtips. My size twelves looked puny as they confronted his massive clodhoppers.

He bent forward, sticking his bright red nose within an inch of mine like an irate baseball manager about to chew the head off some hapless umpire. His eyes squinted in rage. His breath reeked of stale bourbon and cigarettes. "You call yourself a goddamn doctor?" he bellowed. "You're not here to tell us she's gonna die! You're here to get her better."

He pivoted on his heel and lurched toward the door. Once again, my mind stopped, this time in confusion. I was certain that letting him get out that door would be a terrible mistake, even worse than pulling the family together in the first place. So I said the first thing that entered my mind. "Sir, I'll listen to anything you have to say. But please don't leave."

He stopped, silhouetted in the doorway, and swayed slightly. Then he turned, stumbled back into the room, and slumped down on the bed, scattering the little farm animals as the grandkids shrieked. At that point, he burst into tears.

I was happy that everyone was focused on him, because I had no idea what to do next. *What a disaster. This is what I get for poking my nose into family business.*

Without warning, a couple of family members rose out of their chairs and advanced toward me. I wondered how I could possibly defend myself against this mob. But instead of attacking me, they smiled and reached out their hands. "Thank you, thank you!" they cried.

My mind reeled. *For what!?*

One of Mrs. Dinucci's sons grabbed my hand and shook it. A daughter gave me a hug. Others gathered around, all chattering. Piece by piece, the family story emerged.

The man sobbing on the bed was Mrs. Dinucchi's ex-husband. No one had seen him for years. When he heard about her cancer, he drove across the country without calling ahead and just showed up, demanding that every possible medical measure be applied to save his wife.

As I would come to learn, this was an extreme version of a common scenario: the estranged family member returns, his guilt at abandoning the patient moving him to demand she be cured.

In this case, Mr. Dinucci had taken the entire family hostage by the sheer force of his personality. Many of them understood and agreed with Mrs. Dinucci's decision to forego further treatment, but the forbidding presence of her ex-husband had precluded any discussion.

Mrs. Dinucchi's ex was the branch that needed to be removed from the logjam to open the way for her wishes to be met. Fortuitously, the family meeting had allowed that to happen. I shook my head at my good luck. I revised my opinion about my decision-making process, raising it up a notch from dumb to kind of courageous. *And I might still make it home for dinner.*

After a few more minutes of warm conversation, I told the family I would convey Mrs. Dinucci's preferences to my partner and to her oncologist. Then I said goodbye and walked out to the nurses' station to write my note. I left a message with the answering service so my partner would know what happened.

Mrs. Dinucchi was discharged to her home in the redwoods the next day. She died peacefully three weeks later, her family all around—including her ex-husband. His tears had helped lubricate his way back into the family.

Thinking back, I wish I could say that I made a brilliant intervention. But the truth is, I just blundered into doing the right thing.

Sigh. Another Learning Experience.

Lesson 1: If you want to be a healer, you need to let people who are suffering know you're willing to listen. But then, you need to be willing to hear whatever they have to say.

Lesson 2: As Louis Pasteur said, chance favors only the prepared mind. However, it's impossible to prepare your mind for an event like this. Yet—there is a way to be prepared for any event.

You have to discover who you really are. That place in you is ready for anything. And that place in you, that link to the eternal, is where those who are suffering long to connect.

CHAPTER 7

See No Evil

One night, years into my practice, I got a call from John, an old friend. Martha and John had a place out in the country. They shared an idyllic life—until cancer showed up. Once that happened, things moved fast.

Martha was diagnosed when the breast cancer had already spread to her lungs, bones, and brain. She underwent aggressive treatment. Tonight, John told me, she could barely breathe.

I told John I'd meet them at the local emergency room. I phoned in an order for a chest X-ray. It was ready when I arrived. Even a third-year medical student could see how bad it looked.

Martha sat on the exam table. Her head hung down and her chest heaved. Her lips were blue. Even with oxygen running at the maximum rate, she gasped for air. John sat by looking concerned, but matter-of-fact as always.

I asked Martha a few quick questions, including a check of her mental status. She was clear-minded, without any signs of dementia or confusion.

She spoke her words one at a time between gulps of air. "Why . . . is it . . . so . . . hard . . . to catch . . . my . . . . . breath?" she gasped.

"Do you want all the details?" I asked.

Martha was sensitive about her cancer and didn't like to talk about it. But now she was frightened. "Yes . . . please . . . I want . . . to know . . . every . . . thing."

I launched into an explanation of all the clinical issues. The bottom line: because of all the damage to her lungs inflicted by cancer and its treatment, she wasn't getting enough oxygen into her bloodstream. But I might as well have been talking to myself.

"I . . . don't . . . get it," said Martha.

Hmm. What else can I say? Maybe it was too complicated for Martha to understand. But that didn't make sense. She was a teacher who was used to explaining things. "Maybe we should look at your chest X-ray?" I suggested. "It might be easier if you saw everything in the form of a picture."

She agreed. I put the films up on the view box about four feet away from Martha and turned the room lights down.

The view from front to back showed that her heart was enlarged. This could have been due to heart failure caused by weakening of her heart muscle from chemotherapy. It might also have reflected fluid accumulation in the *pericardium*, the sac that surrounds the heart—a condition commonly seen in metastatic cancer. Either or both conditions could cause shortness of breath by themselves.

But that was just her heart. In her lungs sat four large tumors, two on each side. Together, they took up more than half the available air space. The cancer had also spread into the lymph nodes between her lungs, enlarging them so they pushed outward from the center of her chest, reducing her lung capacity even further.

The side view told more of the story. The tumor masses were outlined even more clearly. But she had a more serious problem that hadn't been obvious on the frontal view. Fluid had accumulated underneath both of her lungs, pushing them upward so they couldn't inflate fully. To top it all off, scarring from radiation therapy was clearly visible throughout both lungs. Radiotherapy had killed cancer cells in all her lung fields, but it had also damaged healthy lung, causing scar tissue that was now taking up valuable air space. The scarring also made her lungs stiffer, forcing her chest muscles to work harder to move air in and out.

Other nasty things were possible, but it would take more than a chest X-ray to rule them out. Since the nodes between her lungs surrounded the airways leading down from her throat, there was a chance that those enlarging nodes were squeezing her airways shut. Airway obstruction makes breathing difficult, but it can also cause pneumonia in segments of the lung whose air supply has been cut off. On a simple X-ray, the shadows caused by scarring and pneumonia look similar. Martha didn't have fever or chills, but that didn't rule out pneumonia in someone as ill as she was. Her immune system might have been so weak that she was incapable of generating a fever.

The question of airway obstruction was immaterial anyway, because Martha couldn't be treated. The only way to treat airway obstruction is more radiotherapy, and she had already undergone all the radiation her lungs could tolerate.

In short, Martha had a long list of reasons to be breathless, and I had a lot of uncertainty—not only about those reasons, but also about what to do next. As all of this ran through my doctor's mind, I sifted out the biggest issues and talked to Martha and John about them. Those included the tumor, the fluid, and the scarring—the objects most visible on the X-ray.

Unfortunately, it soon became clear that the term *visible* only applied to John. He nodded as I pointed out each of the details.

But Martha didn't. "I . . . can't . . . see." she said.

I tried again. But no matter what I pointed out on the films, and how much I tried to break it down for her, she couldn't see any of it.

By this time, her face was different too. She no longer looked like a schoolteacher in her late fifties with advanced breast cancer. Now she resembled a sick and innocent child. Even though she was barely able to breathe, she smiled in a puzzled way, as if her inability to understand was somehow amusing, even to her.

The teacher that Martha had once been was no longer in the room.

The three of us talked some more. I ordered Martha a small dose of morphine to swallow, easing her breathlessness without making her sleepy. After I wrote her a prescription for oral morphine, John and I talked out in the hall while the nurse helped Martha get dressed.

John was his usual rock-solid self. "Her time is getting close, right?" he said. "I know she doesn't see that, or else she doesn't want to. It's been like that all the way along. Whatever, I'll see it through with her."

That's the way it sometimes goes with denial. When one person doesn't want to see, another may step forward to help bear the burden. Martha was lucky to have John by her side.

Martha died peacefully at home several weeks later. We held a memorial service at the house, then buried her ashes under the redwoods.

We have nothing to fear but nothing itself. Death seems to represent a fearsome void that many people can't bear to contemplate.

When I was young, I was frustrated by people in denial. I'd think, *When your cancer becomes so advanced that you weigh eighty pounds and can't hold food down or get up and walk across the room, why can't you see the obvious?*

But I was being self-centered. What I meant was: *I have to take care of you. Why can't you decide on something reasonable?*

Denial may sound like simple avoidance, but it's actually a complex mélange of issues. Your role in the drama determines your point of view. Are you one of those doctors who gives chemotherapy for a living, whose denial may be related to their unwillingness to reduce their income? Or are you a patient with your life at stake, so overwhelmed by the enormity of your illness that you're unable to grasp what everyone with experience (e.g. doctors) take for granted as *reality*?

We have to be kind to people in denial. Some of them are not simply unwilling to hear these questions. They are literally unable to hear them, much less give them serious thought.

A number of barriers are arrayed against our becoming aware of our own death. We tend to lump all these together and call them *denial*.

It may be helpful to tease the components of denial apart and look at them separately before we simply assault it. Some aspects of denial are not problems at all. In fact, they may be essential to normal functioning. Others we might do better without.

Denial is hard-wired into the human brain. You make use of it every day. You need it to function normally. This kind of denial is the natural tendency to believe (without having to think about it) that what you wake up to tomorrow will be pretty much like what you went through today. That sense of continuity helps you to meet day-to-day responsibilities without being bothered by constant worry and fear.

Imagine what life must be like for refugees in a war zone where nothing is predictable, even shelter or food, and where every day could be their last, or their children's last. In places where death is common and unpredictable, post-traumatic stress disorder (PTSD) is not just an affliction—it's a way of life. And so is denial. Those who can't manifest it would do nothing but huddle helplessly in a corner.

Denial has both mental and emotional components. As soon as you start thinking about dying, you'll automatically have feelings about it. Brain research tells us that thinking and feeling are not just connected. They are part of the same process. Feelings are a vital part of decision making because our feelings determine our values.

However, when it comes to dying, we tend to repress the feelings. Feelings about the end of life are unpleasant. Our culture worships youth and vitality, and we're phobic about death. We do whatever we can to avoid thinking about it. As a result, most of the feelings we have about our own death are based not on facts but on fantasies, and those fantasies are based on fear.

Because we avoid things that make us anxious, we keep death in the closet with the door closed and locked. Then, when end-of-life situations come up in real time, we're ill-equipped to handle them. Most people are forced to work hard to get over an emotional hump before they can make reasonable decisions about treatment for themselves or for those they care deeply about.

Doctors are people, too, and we have the same issues. We confront them—consciously or not—whenever one of our patients becomes seriously ill. If those emotional challenges remain unexamined, they can have practical consequences.

Doctors tend to overestimate prognosis in their sickest patients, and not just by a small amount. On average, they predict that their seriously ill patients will live up to five times longer than they actually do. These predictions have a big influence on treatment decisions. If we doctors weren't so overoptimistic, we might be more realistic.

Surveys show that doctors don't like to tell the truth about dying to their patients. Doctors freely admit to concealing or distorting the truth when their patient's prognosis is poor because they don't want their patients to lose hope. They conceal the truth the most from the patients they're closest to, the ones they've known the longest.

This tendency is a great illustration of what happens when people are pulled off center by another person's suffering—or the fear that they might cause it.

Ironically, if you ask them, most patients want to know how long they have, and when they're told the truth, they don't suffer from depression or anxiety. On the contrary, they feel more in control, and they make better decisions—ideally in partnership with doctors who are committed to shared decision-making. Yet many doctors are reluctant to go there.

You can prepare yourself all you want, but that doesn't mean you'll have an easy time when you confront your own death. It's all theory until it's real.

Many people believe they've solved the problem of death ahead of time. It's been said, "The fear of death follows from the fear of life. A man who lives fully is prepared to die at any time" (Abbey 2015).

A man who lives that fully might want to be cautious, as he may be possessed by the kind of bravado that crumbles when death actually shows up.

Many people believe they have come to terms with the end of life before they arrive there. That's good if it helps you make decisions in advance about what kind of treatment you want—or more importantly, don't want—if you should grow so ill you can't speak for yourself. That's called Advance Care Planning (ACP). Perhaps the most important component of ACP is to appoint someone you trust to make care decisions for you in case you lose the capacity to make them yourself.

This makes sense. As you move near death, about one-third of the time you'll be too ill, sleepy, or confused to make any plans. If you don't prepare for this, and if you're unable to make those decisions on your own, you'll force others to make them for you. That's a heavy burden for them to bear.

All the notorious court cases deciding the touchy issue of removing someone from life support—from Karen Ann Quinlan to Terry Schaivo—involved people who had neglected to make their wishes known in advance or to designate someone else to do it.

Only rarely can denial be resolved by the brute force of confrontation. A better solution might be to take a long look at the denier and their situation—from their point of view. They may have good reasons for staying in that state of mind, or at least not rushing toward accepting your view of reality.

Some people take a while to find acceptance. But even if that process takes time, they often wind up in a good place.

CHAPTER 8

Her Way

Edie strode into my office followed by her husband Roger and two children, aged three and seven. Her cheeks were sunken from chemo, but her eyes were defiant. Her figure was young and frail. Her thinning hair stood out from her scalp in spikes.

It was 1998. I had been a hospice medical director for about five years.

Edie was here to tell me about her healthcare decisions—in no uncertain terms.

"I've got breast cancer with a year or two left," she said. "When my time comes, I don't want to fight any more. I want to be in hospice."

"Okay," I replied. "How are you going to know when there's no reason to fight any more?"

"Trust me," she declared. "I'll know."

Roger shrugged. "She'll know."

I was skeptical. Edie was a mother with two young kids. It's one thing to confront dying in your mind. But what would happen when reality sank in?

A few weeks later Roger called. "Edie's gotten a lot worse," he said. "The cancer is spreading like wildfire. It's in her bones, lungs, liver, brain, everywhere. It's hard for her just to walk to the bathroom."

"Sounds like it's time for hospice," I said.

"That's why I called," said Roger. "She changed her mind. She's going after every treatment she can find."

"Should we get together again?" I asked.

"Forget it," said Roger. "I tried to bring it up, but she changed the subject."

Edie requested more treatment from the local oncology group, but they refused. She'd been tried on all available chemotherapy, including experimental drugs, and she hadn't responded to any of them. She'd had all the radiation her brain, spine, and lungs could tolerate. A nearby academic center had refused her too. Finally she bought a ticket to Florida where some cowboy with a gamma knife treated over seventy-five tumors in her brain. This would have put most normal people in the hospital for a long time.

Edie recovered in a few days and flew home, but she continued to go downhill.

A week later Roger called again, this time more desperate. "Can you come out to the house?" he pleaded. "It's crazy here. Edie's parents showed up. They survived the Nazi death camps and moved to Argentina. Her dad is a physician. He wants her to get better no matter what. Her mom thinks we should let her die, the sooner the better. It's like World War II all over again. Edie agrees with her dad. But she's so weak she can barely get out of bed."

I drove to their place, a beautiful ranch home on a tree-lined street in the hills above town. Roger greeted me at the door. I sat down with him and Edie's parents.

They were just like Roger described them. Edie's father was adamant that everything possible be done for his daughter. Her mother disagreed, screaming at him in Portuguese, German, and Yiddish. I felt like an onlooker at a street fight.

Finally, Roger led me to a small back bedroom. Edie was propped up on pillows. Her skin was stretched taut over her bones. Scattered wisps of hair clung to her scalp. Her smile was as thin as the rest of her. "Hello, Dr. Stuart," she murmured. "I wasn't expecting you."

"Hi Edie," I said. "I just came by to say hi."

She got right to the point. "I'm not ready for hospice. I don't know. I think I'm getting better."

Roger rejoined Edie's parents. I sat down on the foot of the bed. "So how are things?" I asked.

"Kind of spotty," she replied. "One day I feel good; the next day I can barely move. I finally get something down; it comes right back up. Mornings are hard."

"Hard how?" I wondered.

"When I wake up, I can't tell what I'm going to wake up to."

Muffled shouts could be heard through the door. "We could send some folks out from hospice," I suggested.

"I don't think that would work," she said.

"Do you mind if I keep in touch?" I asked.

Finally she looked me in the eyes. "That would be great."

Roger walked me to the door. I didn't have a lot to say. "For some people, the hardest thing in life is to give up control. Edie is one of those people. It seems to run in the family."

"That's for sure," he said.

Three days later Roger called again. "Edie finally said yes to hospice," he told me. "She hasn't been out of bed in a week. She can barely talk. She's just taking nibbles of food and sips of water."

The next day hospice signed Edie up. That was a relief. I hoped the turmoil would level out, but luck wasn't with us.

Roger paged me a few nights later. Now he was frantic. "You won't believe this," he said. "Our son came home last night from the hospice support group. He'd drawn a picture of an angel on a cloud. At the bottom he wrote, 'This is Mommy in heaven.' I thought it was beautiful. Then he showed it to Edie and all hell broke loose."

"What happened?" I asked.

Roger replied, "She took one look at the picture, fell back in bed, and passed out. Her dad ran in and told us all to clear out. He yelled that one of her pupils was a lot bigger than the other one. He wanted to call an ambulance, but Edie's mom wouldn't let him. So he ran out of the house, jumped in his car, and drove off like a maniac. Then he rushed back here with a syringe full of some drug and injected it into her."

I knew what he was trying to do. Cancer in the brain can cause bleeding, raising pressure inside one-half of the skull. The brain is divided in two by a tough membrane. Each half is a closed space with no outlet for the pressure. The swelling brain compresses the nerve that controls the pupil against the base of the skull. Nerve impulses stop and the pupil relaxes, opening wide, while the other side stays normal.

A blown pupil is a very bad sign. As pressure in the brain continues to increase, it cuts off circulation to the centers that control breathing and other basic functions. Few people survive this, especially when they're so ill with end-stage cancer.

Edie's father had injected her with corticosteroids to reduce brain swelling—a desperate and probably futile move. But, defying the odds once again, Edie woke up the next morning.

During lunchtime, Roger called me once more. "Can you come out again?" he asked. "No rush now. She's sleepy but comfortable." He took a breath. "I finally had it up to here with her parents. I told them to find a hotel room. Visiting hours 6 to 8 p.m. Period."

"Good move," I said.

I drove out later that afternoon. Edie was propped up in bed, waiting. She looked like a victim of the death camps herself.

Her voice was soft and weak. "I'm supposed to talk to you," she whispered.

"What are we supposed to talk about?" I asked.

She remained silent, eyes downcast.

"Edie, how are you feeling?" I asked.

She looked up at me. The light glancing off the bed sheets lit up her cheekbones from below. Her hollow eyes were in shadow.

I pulled up a chair at the foot of the bed. "Why don't I just sit down for a while," I said. "We can talk if it feels right."

We sat in silence. The kids played out in the living room. Outside, a dog barked.

Finally Edie spoke. "I try to look ahead," she said, "but all I can see is a big dark cloud of fear. I can't see through it. I can't talk about it. I can't do this."

"What do you have to do?" I asked.

More silence. Then she looked up. "I'm sorry. Thanks for coming out."

"Nothing to be sorry about," I replied. "I'm glad to be here."

I meant it, and she knew it. "I'd better be getting back," I said.

I slid my chair back from the bed.

But Edie was not done. "Wait," she said. "I want to give you a hug."

"All right," I said. I got up, walked toward the head of the bed, and bent over to put my arms around her.

"No," she said flatly. "I want to stand up."

Her statement stood *me* straight up. "I'm not sure that's a good idea," I said.

Edie's bones were full of cancer, which would have softened them. She hadn't stood for weeks, so her bones would have lost calcium, making them even softer. I'd seen less advanced cancer patients break a hip just by putting their weight on it.

"I don't care," she said. "Help me up."

I opened my mouth to argue but closed it again. No use contradicting Edie when her mind was made up. I slid my right hand behind her shoulder blades and lifted her upper body carefully off the pillow. I put my other arm under her knees. I could feel the artery pulsing behind her leg bone. Slowly we pivoted her body around until her legs hung over the edge of the bed. She weighed seventy pounds at most.

I put her quilted booties on her feet. Then I stood up in front of her.

"I'm a little dizzy," she said. "Give me a second."

I waited. I watched her ribs rise and fall inside her flannel pajamas.

Finally she caught her breath. "Okay, I'm ready."

I reached out and took hold of her outstretched hands. Her knuckles were knobby. I leaned back and let Edie do the pulling. It was slow. The muscles of her arms had wasted away.

Slowly she rose until she stood facing me. I took her in my arms. It was like hugging a little bird. Her bones were like fragile porcelain. I dared not squeeze her for fear she'd shatter.

We held each other for a few moments. Edie sobbed once, quietly. Tears ran down my cheeks too. We both knew this was the last time we'd see each other. Yet we couldn't talk about it. Nor could we say goodbye.

We held each other, partners in despair.

I lowered her back down and swung her legs around until finally her head rested back on her pillow.

She looked up at me. "Thanks," she said.

"Anytime," I replied.

We looked into each other's eyes. There was nothing left to say.

Roger was waiting alone in the living room. "How did it go?" he asked.

"Pretty good," I replied.

"God, I wish she could accept that she was dying," he said. "It would be so much better for her if she could talk about it."

"Maybe," I said. I drove back to town.

Over the next few days, Edie grew weaker and weaker. She stopped eating, then drinking. A group of women friends stayed at her bedside, holding vigil with her as she struggled against letting go. Finally, she slipped into unconsciousness, this time for good.

Roger called me the next morning. "We kept Edie's body here," he said. "It was the right thing to do." They had a choice—Edie and Roger were both Orthodox Jewish and Buddhist. Roger continued, "If you have time, stop by and you'll see why."

I cleared my schedule and drove out to their house. Roger walked me back to Edie's room. "It was a horrible night," he said. "She fought so hard. But just as the sun came up, she lay back and relaxed. It was like she came back into herself. Then she just stopped breathing."

We walked into Edie's room. Her body lay flat on the floor, face up, her head on a pillow under the open window. Maybe her friends had helped her crawl there. Her eyes were closed. A slight smile lit her face.

Roger and I sat down on the floor on either side of her. We each put a hand on one of her cold gray shoulders and gazed at her face. We sat there together, the three of us, for a long time.

Finally Roger spoke. "She always did everything her own way," he said.

"That's true," I agreed.

Then she found a better way. It was a sight worth waiting for.

CHAPTER 9

The First

Zola was my receptionist. My practice was a two-person operation. In my office, she was everything besides the doctor. She was white-haired, sweet, and tough.

Zola and I worked together so long I could tell just from the tone of her voice when something serious was happening. One day, I was just finishing with a patient when she called out to me from up front. "It's the ER," she said. "They have somebody they want you to see."

I said goodbye to the patient, phoned the ER doc, got the story, ordered some tests, and hustled across the street to the hospital. Zola would have to apologize for my lateness over the next hour.

Robert was a thin, well-dressed, and reserved young man, age thirty-four, with fever, chills, and a cough. His white count was elevated. His chest X-ray had been ordered by the ER doc. It clearly showed a right middle lobe pneumonia. For a man in good basic health at Robert's age, that was unusual.

But the X-ray also showed something else. The lymph nodes in the middle of his chest were enlarged. During his physical exam, I had noticed some hard nodes above his collarbone, and in his armpits and groin too. His spleen was also enlarged and hard. Usually I can't feel the spleen, and if I can, it's soft—unless it's filled with something abnormal.

His blood count showed he was anemic. I had the lab run one more test on his serum. An enzyme called LDH was abnormally high. Now I had confirmed what the ER doc had suspected and had told Zola that got her so concerned.

I invited Robert to get down off the exam table and sit in a chair. I sat on a revolving stool facing him, so our eyes were on the same level.

We'd already been through some introductions and talked about his medical history. For reasons I didn't yet understand, he'd left something out—something important. I thought I knew what it was, and I thought he should know about it. But it's not something I wanted to come right out and say.

When you want to get a point across, the best way is to ask the right questions.

I started out with the obvious. "It looks like you probably have pneumonia. I think it will be pretty easy to treat. But it looks like something else might be going on too."

"Oh really?" said Robert. "What's that?"

"Some of your lymph nodes are enlarged," I replied. "Does the word *lymphoma* mean anything to you?"

"Oh, that," he said. "Yes, I've been under treatment for lymphoma for quite a while."

There it is. But that's only the beginning of the story. "Lymphoma can be a real issue for your health," I said. "It's funny you didn't mention it."

"Oh, I just live with it," he said. "My doctors tell me not to worry about it. I'm doing fine."

Until this point, he had made pretty good eye contact, but when he said this, he looked down and frowned.

"Can you tell me something about how your lymphoma was discovered and what kind of treatment you've had?" I asked.

Robert told me he lived in another state. He was here for a few days visiting his sister. Three years ago, he grew progressively more tired and lost weight. His doctor noticed some enlarged nodes and sent him to an oncologist. He was diagnosed with non-Hodgkins lymphoma.

Lymphoma is a cancer of the lymphatic system, which in turn is part of the immune system. A single clone of lymphocytes, the immune cells that fight viruses goes rogue and multiplies more or less rapidly. The faster the replication rate, the worse the prognosis.

As most cancers advance, the malignant cells tend to spread to other parts of the body. In lymphoma, the malignant lymphocytes travel to other lymph nodes. The higher the number of abnormal lymph node regions, the worse the prognosis.

The malignant lymphocytes sometimes spread beyond the lymph system. This further worsens the prognosis. The fact that the patient's spleen was enlarged and hard probably indicated that lymphoma had spread there too.

As had happened with Mr. Crawford, lymphoma can also infiltrate the bone marrow, interfering with red cell production and causing anemia—another poor prognostic sign. To top it all off, a high LDH also worsens prognosis.

There are two basic categories of lymphoma: Hodgkin's disease and non-Hodgkins lymphoma. Hodgkin's is often curable, with a five-year survival rate close to 90 percent. Non-Hodgkin's is seldom curable, and factors like the ones mentioned above are all signals that although treatment may be effective at first, it is now losing its potency.

Robert had been treated initially with radiation and chemotherapy. This shrank his diseased nodes considerably but didn't return them to normal. He was sent to a regional cancer center, where he underwent more tests and treatment. He'd been followed there by a number of specialists for the past year or two. Meanwhile, despite repeated doses of chemotherapy, his lymphoma continued to spread.

The evidence was clear. Robert was showing signs that the benefits of his treatment were waning. A few more questions were in order. "Your oncologists have told you you're doing fine," I said. "How do *you* think you're doing?"

"I don't know," he said. "Sometimes I don't feel too good. I'm getting a lot more tired, just like I did when this whole thing started."

Time to get a little more personal. "That must be hard."

"I guess it is," he said. "But I do the best I can."

"Yeah, I can see that," I said. "You look pretty good. But I wonder— how do you see yourself doing in, say, three months?"

"Gosh, I haven't thought about that. But I have to say I don't expect to feel a lot better."

"So what do you think might happen?" I asked.

"Jeez, I don't know."

"Look, I know I'm asking a lot of questions. If they bother you, let me know. But there's a point to all this."

"Yes, I feel that," he said. "I don't mind talking about how I'm doing. In fact I'm a little curious."

"About what?"

He looked directly at me. He hesitated before he spoke. "I've asked my doctors to tell me more about where this is all going, but they don't seem to like talking about it."

"Well," I said, "it might be good for us to talk a little more about it now, if you're willing. You have to understand, though, I'm a general internist, not an oncologist."

"Of course, but you might still know what you're doing."

"We hope so," I laughed. *Now it's safe to go on.* "It sounds like you might be wondering how well your treatment is working. Are you curious about that?"

Another glance downward. "Yes, I am."

"I have a few thoughts about that, but first I want us to be clear. Whatever we talk about here, you need to take it back and talk to your own oncologists about it. I want to do whatever I can to help prepare you for that."

"Got it," he said.

"Okay then. How much do you know about non-Hodgkins lymphoma?"

As it turned out, Robert didn't know much. So I gave him a sketch of the disease and its normal progression. Translating medical-ese into plain English is very satisfying. But I stopped before all the details about prognosis. "So that's roughly how non-Hodgkin's works," I finished. "Does it all make sense?"

"Yes, thanks," he said. "So where am I with the progression part?"

It's nice when the patient asks you what you want to tell them. "It looks like you're moving down that track."

"Okay." He paused. "Like how far down that track?"

"Well, your doctors have done a great job with your treatment. Your lymphoma is getting fairly advanced, yet clinically you're doing really well."

"That's nice. But by *advanced* do you mean, um, getting toward the end?"

The moment of truth. Time to tread lightly. "Could be," I said. "The lymphoma has spread pretty widely. You can see that."

"Yes, I've noticed. Those damn lumps are popping up everywhere."

"Yes. A couple of your lab tests are abnormal too."

I could see him turning the question over in his mind. He'd been pondering it for some time. Finally he asked, "How long do you think I have?"

The big question. It's so tempting to try to give an exact answer. And it's such a mistake. You want to help that person feel less uncertain. But if you try to make an accurate guess, you'll always be wrong.

"I wish I could pin it down for you," I said. "But I just met you today. I haven't seen you over time like your doctors back home have. You really need to sit down and ask them—and keep asking until you're satisfied they're telling you everything they know."

"That's a good idea. I probably should have been doing that all along."

"It never hurts," I said. "Some doctors are relieved when they find out you want to know the truth. They may have wanted to tell you, but they were afraid they might hurt you instead."

"I never thought about it that way."

We're getting there, but we're not quite done. I asked, "Have you thought at all about what kind of treatment you might want if this thing continues to progress?"

"Well," he said, "I guess I assumed they'd continue what they're doing."

Now it's finally safe to get to the point. "They'll keep giving you this kind of treatment, but there may come a time when it doesn't work so well."

He glanced down again. "I've thought a little about that. And it may already be happening."

"I think you're right. What is treatment like for you now?"

"It's hard. I go through a lot."

"Sometimes going through treatment isn't worth what you get out of it," I said. "Then you might have some decisions to make. That's another thing you'll want to talk to your doctors about. And your family."

Robert heaved a sigh. He got it—all of it.

His pneumonia wasn't severe enough to warrant hospitalization—yet. Hopefully his swollen nodes weren't cutting off airflow to the right middle lobe of his lung, and hopefully his bone marrow was still functioning well enough to put out white cells to fight his infection.

If either or both of those were to go bad, he would be back. If not, he would make it back home.

Since he was going to be in town for a couple more days, I wrote Robert a prescription for oral antibiotics and detailed what symptoms to watch out for. If any of them were to happen, he would need to return to the ER right away.

I got ready to head back to my office. Robert put a hand on my arm. I turned to face him.

He had tears in his eyes. "I just want to thank you. I have five different doctors, and you're the first one who's told me what's really going on."

"You're welcome," I said. "But you already suspected most of it. I'm glad I could help. This kind of conversation is hard. Lots of doctors like to postpone it—but you don't want to wait too long. The sooner you understand what's really going on, the more time you have to prepare."

I thanked him too. I was truly grateful that he was willing to be vulnerable enough to share his fear.

I took off to my office. As I walked back across the street, I thought, *I didn't have to tell him a thing. I just asked questions. He already knew the answers.*

You know when you're becoming a healer. You help someone discover they're going to die, and they thank you for it.

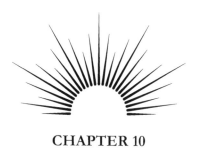

CHAPTER 10

Don't Go In There

I walked into the nurses' station and greeted everyone. It was the start of my week-long shift.

It was 1992. I had closed my internal medicine practice and taken the job of medical director at our local hospice. But it didn't pay enough to support my family. So I became the head of a team of internists and family practice docs in a small rural hospital. We called ourselves Quantum Medical Associates.

In that place, there was too much poverty and too few doctors. It's said that when people fall through the cracks in the San Francisco Bay area, they end up in Sonoma County where I still live today. When they fall through the cracks there, they end up one county north and inland. It's hot, dry, and volcanic. This county leads the rest of the state in only one thing I'm aware of—wildfires.

I liked running this team. In general, I avoided management, particularly of other physicians. It was like picking wild blackberries. Too many thorns and too little fruit, and what fruit there is often turns out to be sour. But on this team of docs, we all got along. Physicians don't do this kind of work unless they care.

Our team took patients who came in through the ER and needed hospitalization, but who didn't have a primary doctor. We cared for them in the hospital until they were ready for discharge, and then we hoped one of the local docs had enough space in his practice—all of them were guys who came on public service grants—to follow the patient.

By chance and necessity, we had become hospitalists before hospitalists were invented. *The New England Journal of Medicine* wouldn't make the term official for four more years.

I was chatting with the nurses that morning, talking over the patients I'd see on rounds. Everything sounded routine until I got to a patient named Kate. She was thirty-two with two young kids. She lived among a large extended family in one of the poorest parts of town.

Or she'd lived there so far. She wouldn't live much longer.

Kate had malignant melanoma that had started on the side of her face. She'd waited to seek medical attention until the cancer had already spread along the side of her head and through the rest of her body. She finally came in to be evaluated and was now recovering from surgery to remove as much of the primary tumor as the surgeon could get.

It wasn't a cure. The cancer was so far along—and her kind of melanoma was so untreatable—that she only had weeks to live. But her surgery had probably served to alleviate some of the suffering she might have faced if the tumor was left alone.

The nurses in this hospital had seen a lot. Their tolerance for behavioral problems was pretty high. But Kate's behavior was difficult even for them. One of the nurses, who was usually polite and reserved, stepped out of character when I asked about Kate.

"Don't go in there, Dr. Stuart," she exclaimed. "That patient is nothing but trouble. She's like a horrible two-year-old. She screams at us. She won't cooperate with anything. She's a total bitch."

I was always attracted to cases like this. Medical problems, after you've seen enough of them, tend to fall into certain categories that, after a few years, feel kind of shopworn. The strategies for handling them are standardized.

I could see it coming. In a few years, there would be clinical guidelines for most diagnoses that every physician would need to follow—or risk having penalties levied against their salaries. Not much room for creativity there.

Sure enough, once those guidelines were implemented, many physicians resented being told what to do. On the other hand, those guidelines moved us past the *Whatever you say, Doc* era. So on balance they've been a good thing.

Even though we didn't have clinical guidelines yet, I was already weary of the routine nature of diagnosing and treating disease categories. That was one reason why I decided to go into end-of-life care. As people near the end of life, you can never tell what's going to happen.

That's especially true of behavioral issues. When seriously ill people act out, there's usually a reason—or a set of reasons as emotional upheaval has any number of causes.

Figuring those out is always challenging. But doing the figuring just challenges the mind. You need to be engaged with people on deeper levels than just the mental one if you want to help with healing.

As I walked toward Room 112—one of only two private rooms in the hospital—another nurse named Barbara met me halfway. She was the hospital discharge planner. Kate was just stable enough after surgery that Barbara could start preparing for her to go home.

It was clear that Barbara felt differently about Kate than the floor nurses did. She seemed to give Kate more space. "I checked the Quantum schedule and saw you were coming on today. I prepared Kate for your visit. I'll go in there with you."

Kate eyed us suspiciously as we walked in. She sat propped up on pillows. I sat on the bed by her feet, and Barbara took a chair.

It was almost hard to look at Kate. The surgeon was forced to remove a large part of her left cheek and half of her ear. She required frequent dressing changes, and blood still soaked through her bandages.

I started at the beginning. "How are you doing?" I asked. It's so easy to make that a throwaway question, but I really wanted to know.

Kate had no trouble answering. She spat out the words. "Fucking horrible." She squinted as she talked. That was a signal.

"Are you having pain?" I asked.

"Am I having pain?" she screamed. "Are you serious? I'm having the worst goddamn pain I have ever experienced in my whole fucking life."

She stopped to take a breath and grimaced. Then she started in again. "And *you* people won't do a fucking thing about it!"

Well. That didn't take long. There were a lot of problems here, but Kate just put her finger on the big one. And we could do something about it.

I asked her a few questions about her pain. She had two different kinds. One is called *somatic*—it resulted from surgical damage to the skin and muscles of her face. Somatic pain happens after any surgery. Kate was receiving medication for that, although the dose was too low.

The other type of pain she had was less common. It's called *neuropathic*. There are many nerves running through the face, and the surgeon had been forced to cut several of them to debulk the tumor. Neuropathic pain is harder to diagnose, often overlooked, and thus often undertreated—or, as in this case, not treated at all.

When you put somatic and neuropathic pain together and fail to relieve them, you have serious trouble. This was the fifth day postop, and Kate had been in severe pain the entire time.

Pain does dreadful things to the brain. First the pain centers light up, then after a short time, other brain networks become activated. It's called recruitment. Those other brain centers regulate sensation and—very relevant in this case—emotion. Untreated pain can trigger unforeseen complications like depression or rage. And rage had apparently been an issue with Kate long before her cancer or her surgery.

Other variables were also in play. Kate was not stupid. She knew how advanced her melanoma had become, and she was aware she had waited too long to get it looked at. And she knew that before long her kids would no longer have a mom.

Physicians often avoid difficult conversations like the one we were having. When doctors are surveyed about this, they tend to respond that they don't like to start these discussions because they take too much time.

That response doesn't hold much water. Within ten minutes, we had gotten to the bottom of Kate's major problem. It doesn't have to take forever. When doctors avoid difficult conversations, it's usually due to factors other than lack of time.

Physician, heal thyself.

Once Kate understood that we were on her side and that we had some ideas that might help, she relaxed. I walked back to the nurse's station and told the staff that things might improve. Then I wrote orders for two different pain medications, one given through an IV pump and the other by mouth.

Within an hour or two, after a couple of upward adjustments to the IV rate, Kate was much more comfortable. And grateful, which was a pleasant surprise to the nurses.

Barbara proceeded with the discharge plan. Kate went home several days later. Hospice visited her there, and her family pitched in to help with her care and her kids. She died, peacefully and in comfort, a few weeks later.

Every situation like this is a potential Learning Experience on the road to healing. All doctors practice at medicine, and some practice at healing. When both are done right, they begin to flow together like two streams making a great river.

This kind of learning only happens when you let yourself care, open up, and listen. Even if you're afraid you won't like what you're going to hear—listen anyway. If you're lucky, you can help. Even if there's not a thing you can *do*, you've already performed the most powerful first act of healing.

> Every act of healing is an act of love.

You've let someone else know you heard them. That means you care. It's an act of love.

That's another thing besides death that we never talk about in medicine. Even though it's what brought many of us into this line of work.

Every act of healing is an act of love.

Today, physicians have terrible problems with compassion fatigue and burnout. Many feel that they can only care so much before their well runs dry. Especially the deep kind of caring required when they're working with someone who's dying and afraid.

There's a secret to avoiding burnout: You don't have to generate that love all by yourself. You can open up to the One Life that runs the universe through love, and let it come through.

It takes very little effort to do that. You locate yourself inside that place where you are who you really are. You might think that you just need to be yourself, but it's not that simple. In fact, it may take effort and time to learn how to get your self out of the way so this love and caring can flow. That's why they call it practice. Don't worry if this doesn't seem clear now. We'll talk more about it in Part II.

It wasn't just my efforts that counted with Kate. I had Barbara's prep work to build on. Barbara was empathic, experienced, and unafraid. Those are all vital qualities. That's not just my professional opinion—it was personal too.

Barbara and I worked together with many other patients. It turned out that we were kindred souls. Years after this, she became my wife.

CHAPTER 11

Bedrock

Pain is physical. Suffering is more complex. It's a multimodal experience, involving the body, the mind, the emotions, and the spirit. Suffering may be a response to simple physical pain, or it may be a reaction to death, loss, damage, disability, or any number of other hardships.

People don't just experience suffering—they endure it. It's an ordeal.

> Pain is physical. Suffering is more complex.

We'll focus on suffering in response to the threat of death here. For convenience, we'll focus on mine.

When I turned fifty-five, I had a physical exam with my primary doctor. Although it wasn't routinely recommended, I requested that a PSA (prostate-specific antigen) test be added to my labs. There was no particular reason for this, except that prostate cancer is somewhat more common among people like me who have done a lot of barbecuing.

My PSA came back positive, although the level was fairly low. We had the test repeated every three months, and my PSA level climbed steadily. Within a year, it had reached the value that triggered biopsy. The biopsy also turned out to be positive. I had prostate cancer.

Many patients have told me that getting a cancer diagnosis is like having a bomb go off in your living room. They're right.

Except my cancer diagnosis didn't just blow out the windows and wreck the furniture in my comfy and secure little figurative house. It made a crater that destroyed the floor and took out the foundation. The effect on my mental and emotional state was overwhelming. I had to take a week off work.

Finally, I got to feel what my patients feel. I'd assumed I had *the death thing* wired. I'd experienced so much, I just assumed when my time came, I'd be able to accept my own mortality with equanimity.

Not so. I was a fool. And like any other fool, I never saw it coming.

You can't know what will happen when you reach that moment of truth. You just don't know how you're going to feel or what you're going to think. For me, it was as simple as it was surprising.

My body had betrayed me. I couldn't believe it. I'd been vigorous all my life. I'd had injuries and major surgeries, but my body had always bounced right back. I could count on it.

Now my body was my enemy. All on its own, it had manufactured something that could kill me. Not just could—*would*.

There was no way to know if the cancer had already spread beyond the capsule surrounding my prostate. No imaging study at that time could reliably show it. And if even one cancer cell had gotten outside, that was it. There were hormone blockers to slow down the progression, but once prostate cancer spreads, there's no cure.

The fear and dread came in waves, without warning. I couldn't screen those feelings out, no matter how hard I tried. I distracted myself—with work, wine, the usual things—but as soon as I let my guard down, the fear and dread came charging back.

One afternoon during my week off, I was sitting in my home office chair on the edge of despair. Finally I decided to stop fighting the feelings. Why not? I couldn't do any worse.

I leaned back and gave in. For a while, all the panic and horror flowed through me, in one end and out the other. Then, once I stopped trying to hold those feelings back, they started to change.

This is what emotions are all about. *E-motion*—feelings change constantly. That's their nature.

I'd been holding onto them, trying to stay in control. That just slowed them down, so they hung around longer.

I remembered all those times when I'd squash my feelings and move my awareness straight up into my head, where I could think my way out of whatever jam my patients or I might be mired in. Then I thought, *this is how I've been handling unpleasant feelings my whole life.*

I always made sure I got to them before they got to me. I threw them in a cage in the basement. Then I ran back upstairs and stuffed towels around the cellar door so I couldn't hear them howling.

To be honest, that's a big reason why I became a doctor—to be in control. If there's a better way to stay in control, I don't know about it.

But cancer is a different kind of wild animal. No wonder its symbol is the crab. It grabs hold of you and won't let go—and not just the parts of your body where it started or spread to. Cancer gets a death grip on your entire self. You can't break free, no matter how hard you try.

It rubs your face in the coldest, hardest fact of your life: At some point you'll be taken.

And you will have nothing to say about it.

That day as I sat in my home office chair, I wasn't thinking any of this. I was just sitting, getting quieter and quieter inside. I wasn't trying to meditate, or concentrate, or contemplate, or any of those things humans do to quiet their minds.

I wasn't trying to do anything. Or think anything. I was just giving up the struggle. All my life I'd struggled and pretended everything was fine—to everyone else, and to myself. But this was different. Struggling was useless.

Then I sank through the floor.

I was still sitting in the same swivel chair, but I was moving downward slowly, at the rate of a foot or two each second. It was as if I was descending down the center of a deep well. I could see clearly. There were cold stone walls all around, laid in a circular fashion. The walls were not far away, maybe four feet in any direction. They were too far away to touch, but I had no urge to reach out. I could see moss growing on some of the rocks. After a while it got darker and cooler. Then there was no more moss.

The deeper I went, the more moist the walls became. It was like being in a cave. There was a smell of wet stone. I could hear water dripping. Each drop echoed slightly. There was no obvious source of light, and the rocks were dark. But I could still see, even after the light above had faded away.

I kept dropping like I was sitting in an elevator. Going down. Finally the wheels on the bottom of my chair clattered as they met the stone floor. I was in a chamber completely lined with dark wet stone. The sound of water dripping was louder. I thought I heard a small stream running somewhere. There was a cool breeze and the air smelled fresh, like spring.

The chamber seemed to extend off to my right, and there was a little more light in that direction. But I felt no need to go there. I just sat in my chair, with no impulse to move. There was nothing else around, just me and the rocks.

It felt good to sit there. Reassuring, comfortable, and safe. I felt like part of a community, even though there seemed to be no beings around. It was like the rocks were living things. They didn't move or make a sound. They were perfectly satisfied just sitting there stacked together.

I felt welcomed, as if my arrival had been expected.

I sat in that place for a long while, although in real time it might have been just a few minutes. Then without warning, I began to rise up again, cruising slowly back up the way I came. In a short time, I rose back through the floor. Once again, I was sitting at my desk.

It would be nice if I could say I'd been transformed by some great revelation. But no, I felt pretty much the same as before. And yet, some whiff of that feeling of community, knowing those dripping rocks were alive, and getting my own personal taste of pure despair and finding it not as bitter as I might have expected—those things stayed with me.

Men with prostate cancer face a lot of treatment options. I decided on radical surgery. The details aren't important, except for the pathology report: There was just one small focus of cancer in my prostate, located very near the capsule but not protruding through it. And that little chunk of cancer was more aggressive than the biopsy had indicated. In other words, I had a close call.

You might think you're prepared to die, but be careful—your preparation might just be from the eyebrows up. It's hard to be fully prepared in your gut for that moment when death actually stares you in the face.

Don't let anyone tell you they know all about death. No one knows until they get there.

I can't say that I know even now. I can't even tell you how I'll react the next time I hear I'm going to die. Unless I die suddenly, I'll certainly hear that sooner or later. But next time, it might seem a little less like a tragedy and a little more like an adventure.

> ## Don't let anyone tell you they know all about death. No one knows until they get there.

Maybe I descended to the level of my own bedrock. Maybe, for me, there's not much lower to sink.

Only time will tell.

CHAPTER 12

We Are Like Ants

I walked into Stephenie's room, wondering if the rumors were true.

I had known her for several years. She had been my wife Barbara's business partner. They had taken over the home health agency at their hospital. The staff loved them both.

Barbara was a good manager. And Stephenie was the perfect partner— solid, dependable, and great with people.

Then she got sick.

I hadn't seen her in a while. I was visiting her now to see how she was doing and because I heard she had a request of me.

Stephenie had been diagnosed with a rare bone cancer in her lower leg. The tumor spread rapidly despite treatment. When metastases appeared in her lungs and the bones of her neck, her oncologists decided to switch to even stronger chemo.

Stephenie traveled to a larger hospital out of town and stayed there a week at a time to undergo chemotherapy. In the middle of one of those sessions, she had a major seizure while she was walking to the bathroom. She fell and hit her head, losing consciousness.

After she woke up, Stephenie told her physicians that she was done fighting the cancer. She just wanted to go home. Her family picked her up and drove her there.

What she didn't tell them—or anyone else—was that when she awoke, she found herself in a very different place than she had been before the seizure.

Stephenie had a husband and two teenage daughters. The family went to church sporadically, but nobody took religion very seriously.

Spirituality, on the other hand, was a high priority for Stephenie. Before her seizure, she had read spiritual books, a paragraph at a time. Then she'd stop and try to digest what she'd learned. It was a slow process.

Stephenie found it hard to talk to her husband about her spirituality. He'd been raised in a strict Baptist family, and when he moved away from them, he left the church behind too.

He pooh-poohed Stephenie's spirituality, so she didn't talk to him about what had happened during the seizure. She didn't talk much to her daughters about it either because she and her husband had decided not to burden the kids with too much talk about the cancer.

But one day, when their father was out of earshot, Stephenie mentioned to her daughters that while she was unconscious after her head trauma and the seizure, she found herself traveling down a dark tunnel toward a bright light. Just like in the movies, she said.

Stephenie got some relief from her pain in their hot tub, but one day she fell and needed help getting out. Although she hadn't fractured anything, the pain worsened. Any movement became hard to tolerate. So she quit work and took to bed.

She enrolled in hospice. That helped her pain. She declined slowly. Her family took turns sleeping on the couch in her room.

According to her daughters, Stephenie became *more* spiritual. When they would worry, Stephenie, always calm and relaxed, would tell them everything would be okay. They remember their mom taking more care of them than they provided to her.

A month or two before she died, Stephenie started having conversations with people who seemed to be up near the ceiling in a corner of her room. No one else could see or hear them. Stephenie did more listening than talking and seemed to agree with most of what her invisible visitors were saying to her. And she laughed a lot. Her daughters asked Stephenie who she was talking with.

"Oh, just Mom and Dad and a few other people," she said.

All those people had died years before. As she got nearer to the end, Stephenie lapsed into a trance much of the time. Her conversations with Mom and Dad and the other people got longer and longer. Her daughters could tell she was getting closer to death when she couldn't concentrate on her favorite TV show, *Touched by an Angel*.

Stephenie's friends—who were also friends of mine—and Barbara all told me that, spiritually speaking, Stephenie was in a special place. I was intrigued. It's common to see people undergo spiritual transformations as they near death, but I'd never seen anyone be transformed weeks or months before.

Stephenie seemed to be breathing some pretty rarefied air. So I paid her a visit. Two visits, in fact. I wanted to know for myself if the stories were true. And I wanted to see if she was doing what so many other dying people try to do when others are around—taking care of them by putting on a good face.

My last visit was a couple of weeks before Stephenie died. I pulled a chair up beside her bed, positioning myself so she wouldn't have to turn her head to see me. I said hi and asked how she was doing.

"I'm fine. I'm happy with who I am," she said.

That was an odd way to start out. I asked her what she meant.

"My forty-six years have gone by in the bat of an eye," she said. "But that's perfect. And it makes me treasure my life even more. I've only had a short time, but I feel good about where I am."

I wondered if she was upset about leaving so soon.

"I've never been mad," she said. "I leave that to my family and friends."

I asked if she had any advice for others in her situation.

"Find joy in whatever you experience," she said. "Even if you have to look pretty hard."

I asked what she did to find that joy.

"There's a place in me that receives," she said. "The weaker I get, the bigger that place gets."

I asked her if she thought that was a spiritual place.

"Oh yes," she answered. "I read spiritual books. Two paragraphs used to be all I could absorb. Now the words just flow into my soul. They're outlined in brilliance."

I asked her what happened when she had the seizure and hit her head.

"When I woke up, I knew I was in another place," she said. "It's the *knowledge place*. I know so much more than before. It's not knowledge from here. It's from that other place."

I asked her whether she could say what that knowledge was about.

She said, "I know I was in a place where love is the most important thing." Then she said something that has always stuck with me. "We think we're so smart. That's not true! We are like ants. Running around, just seeing what's right in front of us, bumping into each other. From this place, I can see everyone doing that. This place is different."

I asked her to say more about the knowledge.

"It's different knowledge than we know, she said. "It's not words. It's more like enlightenment."

She paused. "You get lighter," she said. "Wisdom comes out from that other place."

I asked her about enlightenment.

"Enlightenment is living *honestly*," she said. "You don't have to work at it. We all know right from wrong. Look at what *feels* right, not just what your mind tells you, and you'll automatically be spiritual."

I asked her if she had any regrets.

"The only thing I could have done better," she said, "is I could have shared more of the good *and* the bad."

The one thing everyone said about Stephenie was that she was so sweet.

I asked how she felt about leaving her husband and two young daughters.

"Nobody likes to be left," she said. "But they'll do fine. They'll always be cared for."

I asked how she felt about her treatment and deciding to stop it.

"If there was a cure I'd take it," she said. "But I'd never give up this experience for anything. I feel such peace."

Much more was said. Those were just the high points. Before I left, Stephenie gave me her request.

"Would you do my memorial service?" she asked. "I know you'd understand where I am and what I want."

Of course I would.

"Before the memorial starts, I want there to be enough helium balloons so each person has one. Then have each one write a message of love on a piece of paper and tie it to their balloon. I want you to say a few words about me. Then I want you to go around the group and have everyone say something if they feel like it. Once everyone is done talking, have them all spread out into a big circle. Then when you give the signal, they can all let go of their balloons at once. I want those messages of love to go as far as they can."

As she got closer to death, Stephenie had seizures more and more often. They were difficult to control. I wasn't involved in her care, but if I had been, I'd have had some ambivalence about suppressing her seizures. I would have had to sedate her enough to make her unconscious in order to take the seizures away.

Because Stephenie could no longer express herself at that time, no one could know what she experienced during those seizures. It could have been agony, or simple unconsciousness.

Or bliss.

We held her memorial six days after Stephenie died, on a hilltop overlooking a huge lake. It was a crystal clear October day. The sky was brilliant blue. There was a slight breeze. The crowd was large. Everyone wrote out their message of love and attached it to the ribbon on their balloon.

I said a few things about how hard Stephenie worked to prepare for her knowledge. And that finally she just let go and received it. I thanked her for helping us, the ones who still had more work to do to get to the knowledge place.

As we talked about her, Stephenie's presence seemed strong among us. Then we spread out into a huge circle, just as she'd instructed. I raised my arm, then let it drop.

All at once, 250 balloons, each with a ribbon and a message of love at the end, rose together into the air. Someone started shooting photos. All they show at first is a huge row of balloons extending out on both sides from where we stood. When they got about 100 feet off the ground, the balloons were in a perfect circle.

As they rose further, a strange thing happened. Maybe it was the breeze. Maybe it was Stephenie.

The balloons formed a perfect heart in the sky.

Everyone laughed with joy. Nobody was surprised. We all knew Stephenie was loving it.

The balloons kept rising until we couldn't see them anymore. They'd come down sometime, scattered over miles and miles, spreading the message of love that Stephenie discovered in the knowledge place.

Stephenie was gone, but she wasn't done yet. In 2009, thirteen years later, her oldest daughter's first baby was due. But she went into labor ahead of schedule. Her son was born seven weeks early, small but healthy—on Stephenie's birthday.

Her daughter still cries when she talks about Stephenie. "But it's okay; they're good tears," she says. "My mom really helped me. I'm not afraid of death now. It's as beautiful as birth."

Her daughter became a nurse. "I wanted to give back," she says. "But for a long time, I wasn't ready for the big step."

Then, five years ago, she began working in hospice. Stephenie would love it.

PART II

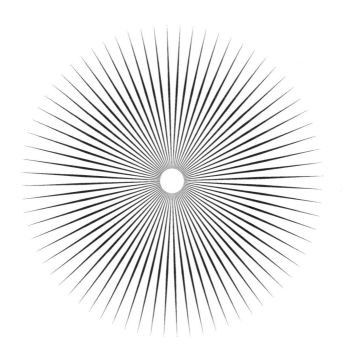

KNOWLEDGE

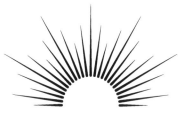

CHAPTER 13

Arrival

It was 10 p.m. on a winter night. The ER was quiet. As is usual late at night, I was the only doctor in this hospital.

Then a young guy threw the door open. A green Volvo station wagon was parked outside. "My wife—she's pregnant!" he cried. "Her water broke!"

Lucia ran out to the car. Carl pushed a wheelchair out the door. He rushed back in wheeling a young woman, pink nightgown stretched tight over her belly. Her long brown hair spread over a puffy blue jacket thrown over her shoulders. She was panting hard.

Lucia helped her up onto the exam table in the main treatment room. She had already taken the history. "This is Maria, twenty-four years old, uneventful pregnancy, decent follow-up, echo normal, this is her third, no major medical problems."

All good. But once a woman gets to her third birth, things can happen fast.

Maria knew this. "I'm close. I wanna push," she panted.

"Let's get you up here safe," I said. "Keep breathing just like you are—you're doing great."

Sure enough, when she was in position, the baby's head was already crowning.

"Okay Maria. Time to push," I said.

The forehead emerged, then the eyes, the nose, the chin. *Bad news.* The face was blue. Not dark blue yet. But still.

"Looking good, Maria," I said. "Push hard. Push-push-push!"

The neck emerged. The umbilical cord was wrapped around it—twice. That's what was cutting off circulation to the baby from the placenta—hence the blue face.

Progress slowed as the shoulders went through the last part of the birth canal. Finally the right one poked out. I was starting to get nervous. Lucia, normally unflappable, was yelling for Maria to push. *Come on baby, come on!*

There, the other shoulder popped out. The rest of the baby slid out fast, like a wet fish swimming in blood and amniotic fluid. "It's a girl!" I said.

My left hand held her neck and upper back as she came out. I cradled her tiny butt in the palm of my right hand and swung her around, sitting her in my lap so I could unwind the cord from around her neck. I left some slack in it so the blood could start to flow.

We were face to face, inches apart. Then it happened.

She opened her eyes.

Little brown eyes in a blue face. Her gaze darted from left to right. She was looking for something. Her eyes met mine. That's what she was looking for—another pair of human eyes. But she was looking for more than that. She wasn't just looking at my eyes—she was peering deep into me. Her brow furrowed. She was very aware and very focused.

As for me, I was transfixed. And transported—to another place. It was strange, but comforting and familiar at the same time. I had no words, no thoughts—in fact, no mind. Just a feeling of astonishment and joy.

Time stopped. I tasted eternity.

Then I snapped back to this world, the one where I was a doctor. That whole interchange lasted a second at most, and nobody noticed it but me.

The baby won't remember. Her brain was far too young to establish memories. Yet in that moment, she certainly registered our encounter. I was privileged. I was the first human to welcome her to this place.

I eased the umbilical cord up over her head. In a few seconds, she pinked right up. Lucia wrapped her in a warm blanket and placed her into her mom's arms. I examined them both. They were perfect. As close as you can get on this planet, at least.

I shook my head to clear it. Then I started in on the paperwork.

Once again, the night was quiet.

CHAPTER 14

Emptiness

I finished the paperwork. One new citizen, duly registered on the county rolls.

But I couldn't stop thinking about that look in her eyes. Searching—curiosity—satisfaction at making contact. I was sure my mind put its own spin on her gaze. On the other hand, I remembered clearly what was in my mind when she opened her eyes and looked into mine.

Nothing!

When her mom was in position and the birth was already in high gear, seemingly an eternity ago, I was focused but calm. My mind was engaged. On a scale of 0 to 100 mph, I was doing about 40.

Birth is a natural process. In general, you don't have to mess with it. You stand by, stay alert, and lend all possible support to the mother. You keep an eye on the details. If there's nothing to worry about, you just go with the process.

That changed in an instant once the baby's blue face emerged. My mind jumped straight from 40 mph to 120, screaming at me as it raced in high gear, gas pedal jammed to the floor:

She's blue, short on oxygen, she's not dark blue just moderately blue, what could be the cause, got to get her chest out of there so she can grab a breath and fill her lungs, c'mon mom PUSH, damn I hope the problem is something simple, we're out here in the boonies and I have no backup, what if we can't stabilize her . . .

Then her eyes popped open, and she nailed me with her gaze. It was as if somebody killed the ignition. My mind turned off. No thoughts.

Instantly, I was empty. Just *there*. With her. I forgot myself. It didn't feel strange. In fact it felt more normal than normal.

Funny, I've been here before, although I can't remember when. It seems like a long time ago—if time has any meaning in this place.

I didn't have glorious visions. I didn't have anything. It was like somebody pulled the plug in the bathtub. Every thought that had filled my head a moment before instantly drained away.

I'm empty. A void.

Her brown eyes didn't move. I stared into the blackness of her pupils. She did the same with me. Except it wasn't she and I. It wasn't even *we*. We were One. One Life.

Wherever she came from, she was still connected there, and I was connected through her. That One Life still filled her through some kind of invisible connection, back through the portal she emerged from.

All that flashed through my mind in less than a second.

Whoa, wait! Back to earth!

I inserted my gloved index finger under the earthly umbilical cord, the one that connected her with her mother, and slid it up over her head. Within seconds, her circulation was functioning normally.

She had arrived. She was safe. I was left with the paperwork. And once that was done, I was left with my thoughts.

That was thirty years ago. It takes a while for the dust to settle.

CHAPTER 15

Awakening

Zen monks can wake you up with a koan, a saying that stops your mind so reality can shine through. Sages from India can touch you between your eyes, stun your mind, and awaken the *kundalini* energy at the base of your spine, shooting it up and out the top of your head, revealing your spiritual energetics.

Then there's Laozi (*Lao-tzu* in the older system of Chinese transliteration), the aged Chinese librarian who lived in 600 BCE. Confucius knew him and consulted with him.

Legend has it that Laozi grew so disgusted with the moral decline in his home kingdom of Zhou that he left town and traveled north to become a hermit. The gatekeeper at the border, Yin Xi, recognized him and would not let him pass until Laozi wrote down his thoughts.

The short book that resulted was the *Daodejing (Tao-te Ching)*. Once he finished it, Laozi, not a fan of celebrity, passed through the gate into the wilderness and was never seen again.

The *Daodejing* is a powerful piece of work. It has been translated into English more often than any book other than the Bible.

Laozi describes Tao, or *the way*. But right at the beginning, he takes great pains to state that this most vital essence he's about to describe can't be described.

That's the essence of ineffability. Anyone with psychedelic experience will identify.

Here's the entire *Daodejing* (Lao Tsu, 2012), Chapter One:

> The Tao that can be told is not the eternal Tao.
> The name that can be named is not the eternal name.
> The nameless is the beginning of heaven and earth.
> The named is the mother of ten thousand things.
> Ever desireless, one can see the mystery.
> Ever desiring, one can see the manifestations.
> These two spring from the same source but differ in name.
> This appears as darkness.
> Darkness within darkness.
> The gate to all mystery.

Although the dates are hazy, Laozi wrote this about 100 years before Buddha came to his own realizations about desirelessness, and half a millennium before Jesus preached the mysteries of the kingdom of heaven within. Buddhism and Christianity both have a lot to say about all this.

But if you want to understand who you really are and why it's important, all you need is Chapter One. Let's break it down.

The Straitjacket of Language

The Tao that can be told is not the eternal Tao. You can't express eternal truth in any language—especially English, which is becoming the world standard

(Pueyo 2022). Language is completely earthbound and incompatible with eternal truth. To see why, all you need is your eighth grade English grammar workbook.

To communicate thoughts, you need to make sentences. The rules are clear. You can't break them. Well, unless you're James Joyce.

You remember. Every sentence requires a subject, the agent that performs an action. Then there needs to be a verb that describes the action, even if it's just some version of *to be*. Then comes the object, the thing that is acted on.

Those are the fundamentals. Everything expressed in language must be forced into this mold. Some discrete subject, separate from all other subjects, does something specific to (or just hangs out with) some discrete object.

This works for describing all the events, relationships, and even scientific theories on Earth, including the most profound ones. The limitations of language also apply to mathematics—the only difference is in the format. Instead of subject, verb, and predicate, math requires that each value on either side of the equation be, well, equal. Regardless of whether you're talking math or language, neither one is up to the task of describing the eternal.

Take Einstein's theory of general relativity, published in 1916. It was revolutionary. Overnight, it replaced Newton's law of universal gravitation as the optimal way to explain how the universe works. General relativity was a complete redo of our concepts of the nature of space and time. Among many other things, it predicted that light would be bent by the gravity of massive objects—if they were massive enough, light wouldn't escape at all—and that gravity would be found to move in waves just like light.

Technology finally caught up to Einstein, over half a century after he died in 1955. In 2015, the Laser Interferometer Gravitational Wave Observatory (LIGO) finally detected gravitational waves. The three physicists who founded LIGO won the Nobel Prize—which, ironically, Einstein never did for his theory of general relativity. Today, we're finally seeing the first photos of the massive black hole at the center of our own Milky Way galaxy. Or to be more precise, we're seeing the energy emitted by the stuff swirling madly around the black hole—which, as Einstein predicted, is so massive that its gravitational well prevents any light from escaping.

The fundamental truth of general relativity wasn't expressed primarily in English, or even in Einstein's native German. It was presented as mathematical equations. Eloquent physicists can present us with general relativity in understandable English (Siegel 2021).

General relativity. Scientifically, you can't get much more profound than that. Yet no matter what language you use—mathematics or English—you can't describe anything beyond the edge of the universe, or the edge of time. Relative to us, they're the same thing.

Transcending Time and Space, Right Now

Ironically, language itself, especially writing, transcends time and space by nature. As you're reading this, I'm talking to you *right now*. But I'm not with you physically—we're transcending distance, or space. And when you read this, I might not even be on the planet anymore, so we're transcending time too.

But Laozi knew that what language *is* doesn't extend to what language *does*. Unfortunately, you can't use language to express the *experience* of the eternal.

Nevertheless, my essence is with you no matter what happens to my body. As Jesus said, "I am always with you" (Matthew 28:20). Those two words, "I Am," are crucial.

When Moses asked God to identify Himself during the burning bush conversation, God replied, "I AM that I AM" (Exodus 3:14). He meant that He just *is*, was, and will be, and nothing else matters—so don't bother asking silly questions.

> You can't find the meaning of life by asking questions. The meaning of life comes from inside life itself.

When Buddha was asked questions like that, it's said he remained silent and just held up a flower—because a flower just *is,* and only for now. That's where its beauty comes from.

You can't find the meaning of life by asking questions. The meaning of life comes from inside life itself.

The bottom line: *I Am* is who you are.

The Language of the Void

To the best of our knowledge, the universe originated from—nothing (Siegel 2022).

And, as the ultimate cosmic joke, we've just figured out that *dark energy* is expanding space and time throughout the universe, and that expansion is accelerating. In a hundred million years, our Milky Way will be isolated in space. Even today, the rate of cosmic expansion is so rapid that you could never reach 94 percent of other galaxies even if you traveled at the speed of light—the ultimate speed limit.

It's as if the universe is a puff of smoke breathed into the void, here now and gone tomorrow. Out of nothing, back into nothing.

Cosmic expansion is strange. It's not that the universe is taking up more space. It's that space-time itself is expanding. We don't understand why or how—yet.

Astrophysicist Kate Mack explains it best: "Space is expanding the way your mind is expanding. They're not expanding into anything. You're just getting less dense" (Mack 2020). However, even when we come to understand dark energy, we still won't have grasped the nature of the eternal.

Meanwhile, we speak to each other using language we developed as we evolved from hunter-gatherers into farmers grouped in little villages. Specific subjects performing definite acts on particular objects. That's not a recipe for describing the eternal. You can get fairly close with poetry, or you can use metaphors.

Jesus did a nice job with parables, but there's a reason why in the Old Testament God wasn't allowed to have a name. Because the god who can be named is not the eternal God.

The infinite, the timeless, the eternal—the words are suggestive, they might satisfy your mind, but they can't convey the *experience*.

Any direct experience of the eternal is, by definition, mystical. It's ineffable, indescribable in everyday language. And take my word for it, unacceptable in medical journals. Except maybe in the poetry section.

But one recent and notable exception is in scientific articles about psychedelics. The mystical component of the psilocybin experience is where the therapeutic action is (Chi, Gold 2020). Still, the language is of this world.

I know what you're thinking. If language is so inadequate, why write this book? Or—why read this book? Maybe we're both crazy.

No. It's just life. As long as we're here, we'll never get everything we want. But we'll get as close as we can.

Like cosmic dust swirling around the black hole, we'll snuggle right up next to the void before we cease to exist.

The Name That Cannot Be Named

What's true for language is true for the mind itself. Language is simply distilled thought, formulated in a standardized way so that one mind can communicate with the next.

You can't speak eternal truth by using language, and you can't grasp eternal truth with your mind.

You may discover some miraculous, world-changing principle that alters the course of history. But revolutionary products of the mind, such as general relativity and quantum mechanics—the two most recent paradigm-shifting theories developed since the European enlightenment—only shake the earth.

They don't change, or even define, ultimate reality. As Laozi points out, they have nothing to do with eternal truth. In fact, any true scientist will agree with Laozi. Science carries us as close as the mind can get to describing the nature of physical reality. But, like it or not, scientific truth is always provisional.

Ironically, that's what's so great about science. It's earthbound, yet it yearns to go beyond itself. Once a milestone like general relativity is established and proven within established limits of uncertainty, scientists can hardly wait until some random observation comes along that turns out to be an exception. Then the race is on to develop a better theory—and that still won't cover reality, let alone the eternal.

Today, physicists are intrigued (*tortured* might be a better term) by an inescapable problem. Einstein's general relativity, the most accurate description of how matter behaves at the vast cosmic level, is irreconcilable with quantum mechanics, the most accurate description of how matter behaves at the minutest atomic level. Both theories predict with incredible mathematical precision exactly how the universe works at both the largest and smallest scales. But no matter how many brilliant minds have tried to reconcile them, they refuse to agree.

Maybe some postdoctoral fellow laboring at some university right now will be the new Einstein who comes up with the elusive *theory of everything*. To accomplish that, they may have to alter some of the basic assumptions that science currently takes for granted.

My money would be on a new theory about consciousness and the nature of reality.

Meanwhile, from the eternal perspective, a new theory about how the universe works doesn't matter. If Laozi heard that a new theory of everything had been proven out to Six Sigma (that is, with 99.9997 percent certainty), you know exactly what he would say:

"Eh. So what?"

Or being extremely wise, he'd probably just sit there and smile, just like Buddha would 100 years later. Because they know that the name that can be named is not the eternal name.

A new theory of everything is just a fancy new name, one step closer to the edge of the world—which is the same as the edge of the mind. Maybe 13.8 billion years ago, the big bang was the beginning of our universe and cosmic expansion and cooling have given us our planetary home and we know that's true out to ten decimal places.

So what? The big bang, or any other explanation the mind can come up with, was not the *true* beginning of heaven and earth.

Why?

The Nameless

Because the nameless is the beginning of heaven and earth. Is, not was. Because we're talking eternal—outside of time as our minds conceive it.

The named, on the other hand, *is the beginning of ten thousand things.* Meaning all the things you can see, hear, taste, smell, touch, and, therefore, think about and have feelings about.

And measure. If you can pick it up with your senses or the instruments that extend them, you can measure it. Once you can measure it, you can create theories about it, test them, make predictions, and control the process. That's the sum total of what science is about.

But—you can't measure the eternal.

From my own personal and professional points of view, that's what's so frustrating about scientific medicine. It's a great way to deal with disease down to the molecular level. So many fantastic discoveries are right around the corner. But scientific medicine has no way of dealing with eternal truth.

Why should you—especially if you aspire to be a healer—care about that? Because at some point in your own personal future, you will die. Ironically, because scientific medicine has gotten so good at postponing death through resuscitation science and critical care, you will most likely have time to contemplate the eternal before you depart.

That's what you'll tend to do once you get your worldly affairs in order—assuming you've found some peace and quiet on the other side of the personal darkness that tends to descend upon you when you realize you're going to die.

Scientific medicine can't help you transcend that darkness. Theories don't help, no matter how grand they may be. When you know that you or someone you love is about to die, who gives a rip about theory?

We're talking practical. There's no point in discussing any of this stuff about spirituality unless you can bring heaven down to earth and make it work for you here and now.

Can you do that with the eternal? Of course you can.

The Ever-Desireless and the Ever-Desiring

First you need to understand the difference between the desireless and the desiring, and how they both spring from the same place.

Ever desireless, one can see the mystery. If you're centered in the real *you*, you can see the mystery. Better yet, you can *be* it. You *are* the mystery. And meanwhile, while you're sitting there being desireless, you'll notice that the mystery is no big deal. It's just natural. Ordinary goodness, for which you feel grateful. Or even blissful.

On the other hand, *Ever desiring, one can see the manifestations.* If you're like most people, you walk around pursuing your daily business inside your everyday self—the one that all spiritual traditions try to help you get beyond. Or inside. Or under.

Whatever, it's not really you. It's just an elaborate structure your mind has manufactured, starting the day you were born (conditioned by your genetics) to enable you to get by in this world.

Creating your self is what your mind was born to do.

That baby who helped me wake up is now about thirty years old, undoubtedly living inside her own self, maybe with three kids who are on the same track. That's what we're all born on this planet to do.

That self is ever-desiring by nature. Assuming you value being alive, that's a good thing. If you stopped desiring those things you need to survive, you wouldn't last long. Your brain

> Creating your self is what your mind was born to do.

won't let you stop desiring—not without a struggle at least—unless you've found a way to get beneath your desires, to the desireless place. If you do that, even for a second, you know the way—the Tao.

Looking at things from that ever-desiring place (that the Buddha will later transcend) shows you exactly what it's designed to show you. That place is your self—an entity that will do what works in the world.

That self, ever-desiring, will see the manifestations. They're easy to see. In fact, they're impossible to miss. They're right in front of you, manufactured by your mind.

They come from nothing—their source is a mystery. But once they're manifested, they're made to be used to satisfy your desires. You might be conscious of those desires, or you might not. Those desires may be constructive, functional, *positive*. Or they might be twisted, dysfunctional, *negative*.

Whatever, they will manifest, and the result will have a major influence on your life on this planet. In fact, those ten thousand things you manifest *are* your life on this planet.

It pays to get conscious about your ever-desiring self. Only then can you start to get some control over the manifestation process.

Darkness Within Darkness

Your self will never show you the eternal. You can use all the tools your self has at its disposal—your intellect, your imagination, your feelings—to conjure up a picture of the eternal that's grand and inspiring. But it's just a representation. Maybe, if you're creative and persistent, it's a map toward the way out, but it's never the real thing.

If you're like most people, you assume in every waking moment that your manufactured self is really you. Haha, sorry. It's not.

Believing you are nothing but your self won't prevent you from living a completely successful life by worldly standards. A life that may be satisfying in every respect. Except one. In the darkness of your inner, desireless *you*, you will know you're missing something. You will know that everything you see is just a manifestation of something deeper and more mysterious.

That *something* is enticing. But it's out of your reach. Until you learn the difference between your manufactured self and the real *you*, you will feel the tantalizing presence of the mystery, but you won't *see the mystery*.

To do that, you need to tease apart the ever-desiring—your *self*—and the ever-desireless—the real *you*.

It's confusing, because like Laozi says, *These two spring from the same source. But they differ in name.*

Darkness within darkness. The gate to all mystery.

So, how do you sort them out?

CHAPTER 16

Who You Aren't

When that baby was born and looked me in the eye, she gave me a gift. She reminded me of who I am. I had forgotten. But no shame—we all do.

Who are you? You may not always feel comfortable with your self as a person. You have your issues. But you probably feel no inner conflict when you use the word *me*. You think you know just what you mean.

Humans get clear that they are a real person, separate from everybody else but relating to others as people *outside*, about the age of two. From that point on, when somebody points to you and says *you*, you have a clear picture of what they mean. And when you think *me*, even now, you're focused on that same image.

You assume you know who you are.

What Makes You *You*?

Most people don't spend much time thinking about who they really are. Tim Urban, in his wonderful blog *Wait But Why*, has a brilliant discussion about this (Urban 2014). You might be more confused about *you* than you think.

You might be your body. You've been residing in it ever since you got here. It's how others recognize you when they see you. Of course, a third of a trillion of your cells are replaced every day, and most all of them will be completely different within seven to ten years, so maybe that's not it.

How about your DNA? It stays the same throughout out your life. It's unique to you—unless you have an identical twin. That person won't ever mistake themselves for you.

Maybe you are your brain? But what if you agreed on a brain swap with a good friend? Before you try this, you'd probably want to check to make sure your political views are roughly similar. Assume your entire consciousness is generated by and contained in your brain (although this theory is highly suspect, as we'll discuss).

In your new body, would you still feel like you? Memories, check. Feelings, check. That bothersome belly flab, maybe not. But overall, you would probably still feel like you. In fact, your brain would experience this procedure not as a brain transplant but as a whole-body transplant. You'd have a different body, yet you'd still feel like your self.

Then again, maybe you're not your physical brain. That's just the hardware—although John Wayne and others who have had their brains cryogenically frozen might disagree. They hope to be resurrected once the proper technology arrives.

Maybe you're the sum total of the data stored in there. There's now serious debate about the feasibility of uploading the entire contents of your consciousness and storing it. Then, the theory goes, your consciousness could be downloaded into another brain—with or without a body. You'd have achieved digital immortality.

That idea may sound like science fiction, but it's not new. Transferring all the data from your brain into someone else's is just today's hi-tech version of a very old idea. Enlightenment philosopher John Locke (1632–1704) wrote that you are you because of the contents of your consciousness. That consciousness could be transferred from one "substance," or soul, to another (Nimbalkar 2011).

If you can pull that off, you've swapped souls, but your consciousness stays the same. You may be a different person (or soul), but you're still you.

Are you less confused now about who you are? Maybe not.

This is what happens when you believe who you really are is something physical.

Beyond the Edge

It's not that your mind is somehow inept or incapable of understanding the problem of consciousness and how it relates to identity, the *who are you really* problem. It's that your mind (and its extension, science) can go right to the edge of the problem, but not beyond to the center of it. Your analytic mind can go right to the edge of the world, which is the same as the edge of your thinking.

Because you're single-minded about surviving in this world, going to the edge doesn't feel safe. Your mind will say, *Don't go there.*

You can see this happening in real time on an international scale. Just page through the latest issue of the *New England Journal of Medicine*. The edges of the scientific mind, beyond which you must not go, are very clear. If you're familiar with trying to get articles that go outside the edges published in that journal, you'll know just what I mean.

It won't always be that way. All we need is a new scientific paradigm.

But at this stage of the game, the boundaries are immutable. Your mind, no matter how brilliant, can't help you know who you really are.

Why? Because going to the edge of the world, which is as far as the mind can go (not counting fantasy novels), isn't quite far enough to help you know who you really are.

Because it's right past the edge of the world that the answer lies.

Through the Mirror

The world you live in is bounded by a mirror. Everything you see is a reflection of what you've created. As you look with your eyes, and as you think about what you see with your mind, you will never behold anything beyond the mirror.

As long as you believe only your mind, you're stuck. And as long as you believe your mind's creation—your self—is really you, you're not capable of going past the edge of the world.

Don't feel bad. It's not just your problem. It's everyone's problem.

Yet you'll go past the edge of everything you think you know, beyond the bounds of your self. But only after you deal with your mind and its prejudices, which are rooted in millions of years of evolution of life on this planet.

> Your mind needs a firmware upgrade.

Your mind will be stubborn, but don't worry, it's safe to go past the edge of the world. You won't fall off. You'll be perfectly supported. You just have to accept that you're going where your mind wasn't originally equipped to go.

Your mind needs a firmware upgrade.

You'll invite your mind to climb out of the driver's seat, walk around the car, be seated on the passenger side, and belt in so it can go along and enjoy the ride. The ride will take you to a place where the darkness within darkness is no longer a mystery. It's reality.

It may take your mind some time to adjust. That firmware is quite firm.

Paradox

It's a challenge. Some things seem impossible to resolve. It's like trying to grasp two opposites at once.

For instance, every person you see appears to be a unique individual, separate, disconnected, living on an island where their brain is isolated from all other brains with no apparent means of communication except through the five senses. Yet, in reality, every person is like a wavelet on the surface of a vast, unknowable ocean, each united with all the others in the immeasurable depths of being.

Maybe you've experienced the isolated individual piece more than you have the wavelet oceanic piece. You're not alone—no matter how much your mind has convinced you that you are. In reality, those two disparate images reconcile. They make sense.

Your mind may not accept this right away. It will try hard to understand. Then after a while, your mind will relax and begin to let go. It will stop trying.

There might be a bit of a struggle. Your mind might fear that if it stops swimming, it will sink. Then it will stop swimming, and it will sink. Into darkness.

Under-Standing

Then your mind will understand because it will be standing under, looking at the problem from below with a deeper perspective.

It's interesting—once you arrive there, there's light inside the darkness.

Or if your mind is more comfortable being elevated and going toward the light, you'll be looking at the problem from above, with a higher perspective. No problem with the light there.

Over the edge, standing under, rising above—it doesn't matter. These perspectives seem different as long as you're rooted in this world. But they're all the same to your mind once it stops trying and becomes more comfortable letting go.

How is it possible to know this? If you have enough experience with living in nature, meditation, psychedelics, sitting with people who are dying, or any number of other activities that can help ease your mind over the edge—you already know this.

CHAPTER 17

The You Within You

To penetrate the darkness within darkness, the first thing you need to accept is that the answer lies within you. You won't find it by rummaging through the details of your life. That's because the details of your life are not within you. They're outside you.

The real you, that is. The only thing inside the real you is pure awareness. No details. Your everyday self is completely immersed in those details. Your self believes they constitute your *real* life.

That's the first hint. The ever-desireless resides within the ever-desiring. As Laozi says, *they spring from the same source.*

The second hint is that the answer is simple. It's been right there in the middle of your consciousness for your entire life. You may never have noticed it. Or you may have noticed it and moved on because it's so simple and ordinary that it seems to have no value. It's just sitting there, a seemingly useless fact of life.

It's like breathing. You do it all the time, but it happens beneath your awareness. You don't notice it unless you choose to. You know breathing is useful, but that's just because at a certain age, you were taught you need to breathe air to survive. Prior to that moment, why would you care about breathing or ever bother to notice it?

The secret lying there inside the darkness within darkness is: there are two *you*s. In fact, they are almost the same thing.

But not quite.

You could say one is nested inside the other. They're so closely connected that you'd think they're one entity. Until you look closely. Then you can tease them apart.

These two *you*s are each places within your own awareness. You can work out of—that is, center your awareness in—either one. But working out of one will allow you to let go of all the things you don't need so you can be free before you die. Working out of the other will keep you trapped, and you won't even know it. Until you're on your deathbed.

When you finally get there, you may be glad you did some prep work.

You and Your Self

These two *you*s are the *I Am*—the real *you*—and your **self**.

There are other labels for the I Am, like *your soul* or *your spirit*. But those terms are overused. They trigger so many associations that they're more trouble than they're worth.

The term *self* has its own baggage. The self, according to Carl Jung, is the sum of your conscious and unconscious—in other words, your entire psyche. That's a little broad, and it's hard to work with your unconscious because, by definition, you don't have access to it. It's impossible to define. Your unconscious, for all we know, extends clear through the portal that bounds life at each end, off into the beyond.

Who knows, if you were single-minded and willing to work hard, you might become conscious of the One Life, the ultimate source, the universal consciousness that your brain interprets as matter and energy. They say some sages have achieved *God Consciousness*, which might be the same thing.

But at this point in our discussion, that's aiming a little high. Right now, we're just focusing on your current life on this plane. The task is to discover the difference between your self and who you really are.

Your *self* is more like a combination of Freud's concept of the ego, plus his concept of the superego, with a dollop of the id on top—but boiled down so it's simple. Unlike your unconscious, you have easy access to your self, or most of it anyway.

That Voice

Unfortunately, your self also has constant access to you, whether you want it to or not. It uses that voice in your head—the one that never stops.

Sometimes your self screams at you. I quoted my self screaming at me when I related what went through my head as that baby's blue face emerged. That's your self when you're engaged in a task.

Neurophysiologists using functional Magnetic Resonance Imaging (fMRI) have found a particular network of brain regions that light up when you're focused on performing any task. It doesn't matter if it involves manipulating an object or doing arithmetic in your head. The Task Positive Network (TPN) will be engaged, and it will light up on fMRI. You may have noticed that your self doesn't bother you so much when you're busy. That's because the TPN is in control. It's when you get done with the task and relax that the trouble starts.

When you're not focused on a task, your self can assume a whole array of different personalities: pleasant company, daydreaming companion, stupid nuisance—or worse. The brain network that functions when your mind is at rest, unengaged in any task, is called the Default Mode Network (DMN). Researchers have used fMRI to study your resting brain, when you're not engaged in a task and your mind is wandering. They can see when one of your thoughts ends and you move on to another. They estimate that each day you have about 6200 thoughts (Craig 2022). That's 43,700 separate thoughts per week or 2¼ million a year.

That's what your mind is up to when you're just sitting around, doing nothing. Although you may not be aware of this, you are a fabulous content creator—far more prolific than anyone on TikTok.

At least TikTok is funny. That voice in your head often isn't.

Research findings in this area are quite new, particularly the ones pertaining to DMN function in meditation and on psychedelics. That evidence points toward some kind of universal consciousness underlying all of reality.

The Tenant You Can't Evict

Whether your mind is focused on a task, idling, or at rest, your self supplies you with a narrator that never shuts up.

Imagine you're walking down the street on a beautiful fall day. You're breathing in the crisp cool air and admiring the leaves just turning colors. That's your mind being mindful, just taking note of your surroundings. That's what your mind is supposed to do.

It's so peaceful—until your self chimes in.

Those red leaves are pretty, says your self. *I wonder why they turn from green to red, wait there's a dead one, ugh it's brown already, looks kind of rotten, it's dry and hanging by a thread, the wind is blowing it back and forth, it's getting cold, I should have brought a coat, I always do this, I'm such an idiot, whoa there comes*

Todd, he makes me uncomfortable, I don't feel like talking to him, maybe I should cross the street, no then he'll think I'm trying to avoid him . . .

It's not until you start to become mindful of that voice that you realize how dumb it can be—and how critical. And how destructive, if the superego part keeps going hard and long enough.

It's ironic because your self evolved to help you survive. Your self is what your brain produces to give you feedback that supports you as you learn to navigate through a world that's become far more complex than the one your ancient ancestors inhabited while your brain itself was evolving. Yet your self can make you feel needlessly awful, or even make you consider ending your own existence.

Your *self* is the end product of an evolutionary neurological chain reaction that has played out over millions of years. You were born with a brain programmed to create your self. That's the genetic piece. The developmental piece started out with your parents, then continued with your teachers.

At some point, developing your self is no longer up to your parents and your teachers. Then it becomes your responsibility. As the ancient Greeks remarked, it's useful to *Know thyself.*

Some people never realize that.

Self-Defense

If you watch your self in action, you may marvel at its structure. So intricate, so elegant. You might feel a sense of pride in your work— because your current self, assuming you're an adult, is largely of your own creation. I remember the very moment I realized that my own self consisted almost entirely of an elaborate facade of interlocking defense mechanisms. That was a letdown.

I had to wonder: *What am I defending myself against?* There was only one conclusion: *life.*

Life is capricious, unpredictable, and full of constant change. In other words, uncomfortable. My self believed there were threats out there, and I'd better be prepared. Childhood experience had convinced me that those might not be just idle threats.

> Just living my life, encountering things as they come up, might be safer than I thought.

You can let go of parts of your self, and you may want to, but you can't get rid of your self. If you're still alive, you still need it.

Yet, I've watched many people drop their defenses one by one as they neared the end of life—until they were defenseless. Lo and behold, by the time they were ready to go, they had no fear. They felt completely safe.

Safe? Facing death, the ultimate threat? Actually, yes. That got me thinking:

Just living my life, encountering things as they come up, might be safer than I thought.

I'm sure your self is not nearly as defensive as mine. But you might want to check to make sure.

Finding Safety

The I Am is not occupied with any of the issues that the self obsesses about. The I Am lives at the center—the very core of your awareness. It's the place where you're simply conscious.

The I Am didn't evolve. It's always existed. It existed before the beginning of the universe. How do you know? Because the I Am is a spark, an extension of the One Life that created the universe.

The I Am is empty. If you succeed in stopping your mind, the I Am is what's left. If you learn to meditate, you may learn to live there.

You can't turn the I Am off. It's present before you arrive on Earth, it's within you all your life—all the time you're awake and all the time you're asleep. It witnesses what your mind creates all day, and it witnesses your dreams at night.

The I Am shines out from within you the moment you're born. It looks for another pair of eyes, and it rejoices when it finds them. It's what mothers see when they look into their babies' eyes. And it's what babies are looking for when they arrive here.

It's what I saw in that baby's eyes, and it's what she awoke in mine. Her eyes were just beginning to see, and the I Am was waiting for that. The I Am in her brought the I Am in me back into my awareness.

I have to admit I was startled. I had forgotten. I was asleep—in waking sleep—the way we all operate most of the time. My self was in control, the way it usually is from the time I get up in the morning until the time I go to sleep at night.

I had forgotten what it was like to be really awake, centered in the place where I Am.

The Other Umbilical Cord

Babies need to see that first pair of eyes for two reasons.

The first one has to do with this world. Unlike most of our animal brothers and sisters, human babies are born long before they are fully developed. A newborn lamb pops out of her mother's womb, stands up on shaky legs, and before long, she's frolicking in the sun.

But newborn human babies can't survive their first couple of years without feeding, protection, and *love*. Why? Because our human brain is so large compared to all our animal cousins. If a human baby's brain were fully developed inside their mother, their head wouldn't begin to fit into the birth canal.

As we humans were evolving our oversize brain, there were no c-sections. So as our brains became larger, we started being born earlier in a developmental sense. Today we're born long before we're mature enough to survive independently. Our brain is as small as possible at birth, and then its development explodes. A baby's brain grows so rapidly after they're born that by the time they're three months old, their brain is half the size of an adult's.

So once babies arrive here, they need to see that other pair of eyes right away. Only after their eyes meet the eyes of another human can they feel safe. Where there are eyes, there are warmth, food, and love.

And they will continue to feel safe—to the degree that their mother's (or someone's) eyes mirror back to them the love that brought them here. Lack of mirroring is a form of neglect. If your self developed in an environment where love was not mirrored, you might have issues with anxiety. It's hard to feel safe in life if you didn't experience a safe start.

Re-Membering
The second reason why newborns need to see another pair of eyes is only partly of this world.

It was a long journey from wherever their I Am originated to their life here. As their body developed within their mother's womb, they floated weightlessly in their private sea of amniotic fluid. Their brain and sense organs formed and began to mature. They heard the back and forth of their family's conversations.

They felt the emotions their mother was feeling—whether those emotions were pleasant or not. If they weren't pleasant, that's not necessarily a bad thing. This experience prepared them, and may have strengthened them, for their life in this world.

As they began to adapt to life in the womb prior to their birth, they were still linked to where they came from. But as they began to accommodate to this world inside the mother, their link to the One Life became more tenuous. Their I Am started to dissociate from the Source it had been united with. However, that link—that invisible umbilical cord—still connected them.

When they are born and open their eyes, they look for another set of eyes. Before, they were entirely conscious in the I Am. As they suddenly see with their new eyes, they also become fully conscious in this world. What is the first thing they look for?

By instinct, they seek the I Am in the only place they will find it—in another person's eyes. That night, those eyes just happened to be mine. That was this baby's new connection in this world with the One Life she came from. Soon after her birth, like you and me, she forgot, but at birth, she still remembered. It was pure luck—if there is such a thing—that she looked into my eyes and triggered the I Am in me.

At that moment I also re-membered. At that moment, I reconnected with the One Life I left long ago. Except I never really left. I was still an official member. That's what re-membering is all about. You realize that you're never, and can never be, truly alone when you're living in the I Am.

Of course (sigh) I forgot again. My self took over, because that's what it's designed to do.

You can choose to re-member whenever you want, like I did later in my life. Or you can choose not to. It doesn't matter.

Into the I Am

Whatever you choose, you'll become aware of your I Am again when you are close to death. Everything else, all the products of your mind, thought by thought, will depart from your awareness then. When that process is complete, only the I Am will be left.

You do have other options besides waiting until you die. You can learn to meditate—to relax your self and reside within the real *you*. Or you can just learn to go there. It's not hard once you get the hang of it.

It starts with mindfulness. You practice being aware of whatever you're sensing, doing, or thinking. You become present in your world. From there, it's just about letting go—falling back into the simple awareness behind your mind.

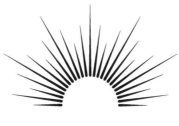

CHAPTER 18

Who You Are

A fleeting moment. A newborn baby looks you in the eye. That moment could have passed unnoticed. But it didn't. It was everything. Maybe I had prepared for it without knowing. But it took me by surprise anyway.

It's fitting that it happened in the emergency room—that place where the miracles of medical technology meet the mysteries of existence. I just happened to have a front-row seat that night.

That night I was gifted with an experience of the I Am, the eternal Presence that exists within you. It's inside you all the time. It's the *darkness within the darkness* that Laozi admired.

Sometimes it rises to the surface so you can experience it directly. So you can see it, feel it, smell it, taste it. Actually experience it. In other words, you can real-ize it. It becomes real, not just some filmy figment manufactured through your intellectual gymnastics.

Real-izing

Language can't express the ineffable. But once you experience the I Am, you see that certain words do *begin* to apply to the eternal.

Self-realization is a term that, like *soul*, carries a lot of baggage. It's been bandied about in spiritual circles forever. Once you offload that baggage, it boils down to this: When you experience the I Am, you real-ize the eternal.

Before that real-ization, the eternal is just a concept. After that, it's real—because every time you center yourself in the I Am, you make the eternal real. You bring it down to earth. You experience it as your own consciousness, your own personal, yet universal, awareness. It's the core of your subjective experience.

> When you experience the I Am, you real-ize the eternal.

That's what the process of real-ization is all about.

Real-ization is no big deal. You don't need all the spiritual inflation, the romanticizing, the glamorizing. You simply bring the eternal into the present. It's literally bringing heaven down to earth.

The I Am is divine, yet it's totally ordinary. It's simply the essence of awareness. It's the *you* that witnesses life. It's the *me* that is always watching, whether I'm awake or asleep.

Here's a symbol that illustrates just how mundane it is. The I Am is that all-seeing eye on top of the pyramid, the Eye of Providence glorified by our forefathers. Traditionally, it's the all-seeing Eye of God, enclosed in a sacred triangle, emanating rays of glory. It symbolizes God watching over all of humanity, all of the universe: God watching from within the universe. God pervading and animating all of the universe. Shining within you and within me. Connecting every atom of the universe into an indivisible, unified whole. Connecting you and me as you read these words. Connecting us outside of time and space.

All right, now let's make it useful. We're talking outside of time and space, but we're talking about it *now*. We're talking Ultimate Value, the only true value.

So let's talk *what's in your wallet*. Yeah, you already know. That all-seeing eye is folded in there waiting to gaze at you off the back of the U.S. one dollar bill.

The Spark

The whole universe is alive and conscious. You can call it God or whatever you want. All spiritual traditions point to the same thing. The great visionaries like Buddha and Jesus realized it and expressed the truth in images, parables, and language that their cultures and traditions had provided them to use.

Now spirituality and science are finally starting to converge so we can all real-ize these truths.

That night the Eye of God gazed at me out of the blue face of a newborn baby. And I sat there entranced, gazing right back. The Eye of God was gazing out of my eyes too. That tiny blue baby sat on my lap, hovering (as we all do) on the knife's edge between the source of her life in this world and the end of her life.

That's why time stopped. We were both suspended in the eternal now, outside of time. That moment lasted forever. Until it passed into the next moment, whereupon it ceased to exist except in my memory. Where it will stay as long as I remain alive on this planet.

Once in a great while, you get to experience who you really are. That's what happened to me that night. I am, just as you are, that pure, silent, eternal point of awareness.

> You are a spark of the One Life that brings this universe into existence in a never-ending stream, from eternal mystery into our finite world of time and space.

The moments of your life pass through that awareness like shining beads on a string drawn through your fingers, or like individual images on film that move just fast enough through the projector of your mind that those present moments appear to blend together into your life.

That *you*, the still point that does nothing but notice, never changes. Every cell in your body will be replaced many times over throughout your life. Yet that *you* remains constant. *Now* and forever—and those two words mean the same thing.

Those moments you experience don't exist at all until you notice them. Once they pass, they cease to exist again, melting back into the void from which they emerged. Those moments only become real because, and only because, that spark of awareness that is the real *you* turned them into reality.

You are a spark of the One Life that brings this universe into existence in a never-ending stream, from eternal mystery into our finite world of time and space.

CHAPTER 19

Damage and the Self

Modern spiritual teachers have captured the difference between the I Am and the self in intriguing ways.

Eckhart Tolle, in his introduction to *The Power of Now*, describes this crucial distinction. At age twenty-nine, he was a graduate student afflicted by a particularly nasty self. He suffered from constant dread and thoughts of suicide. One desperate night, he became obsessed with a single thought: he simply couldn't stand himself.

Suddenly, he realized that there must be two centers of awareness within him. The first was the *I* that was doing the noticing. The second was the self he knew he hated.

Maybe, he thought, *only one of them is real* (Tolle 1999).

That insight stunned him. His mind stopped. And, luckily for him and for us, it didn't start right back up again. He lived in a state of bliss for several months, then read spiritual books and consulted spiritual teachers for several more. He finally came to understand that what the mystics had preached for thousands of years—and what seekers everywhere are looking for today—had happened to him out of the blue.

He realized that who he really was, the I Am, had stopped identifying with his dreary, hopeless self, which was really a fabrication.

Damage and the Self's Reaction

This brings us back to a disturbing but vital observation about the content your mind creates in the process of forming your *self:* that content may be negative, self-critical, and destructive.

The most noxious aspects of your self relate to Freud's superego, the voice that tries to keep you in line. Your self may criticize you whether you deserve it or not. Depending on what kind of parenting you had and how your teachers treated you, your self may be as much of a hindrance as a help.

Say someone in authority had a habit of punishing you physically or emotionally, or completely ignoring you as if you didn't exist. Those two forms of mistreatment are abuse and neglect, respectively. And they can coexist.

Maybe if you experienced those, you were too young to defend yourself. Or if you were young enough, say less than two, you might not even remember them. Either way, life goes on. Assuming you remained alive, you got used to it.

It's really unfortunate when a person becomes so used to abuse and neglect they assume they're a normal part of life.

If you accepted these hurtful events as normal, you internalized them, incorporated them into your self. At that point, your self was trained to treat you the way you were treated. Depending on the quality of your upbringing, that self may be vicious enough to disable you.

When you're deeply immersed in an abusive self, you can lose touch with what's real. Deep depression is a highly malignant form of self-obsession. You can't stop thinking about yourself. It's still creative. It's just all bad.

Christianity gets one thing terribly wrong, and it creates a lot of damage.

You will never go to hell when you die. Hell in the afterlife is a fiction. It was created by religious authorities to keep their followers in line.

Hell in the afterlife doesn't exist. All the evidence we have points to a benevolent and loving experience at death. But hell itself certainly does exist—within your self.

Just this year alone, roughly 10 percent of American adults will suffer at least one episode of major depression, bipolar disorder, or significant dysthymia (persistent and severe low mood). For these individuals, the self-blame and inner torment may seem like hell on earth.

Having been through that myself, I can truly say I never would have believed I had it in me to create something that malevolent. More than once, I said to myself: *So this is where the concept of hell comes from.* It takes a lot of work to dig out of that hole.

That damage reveals its effects not only through your memories, but also through your own feelings, actions, and behaviors. You pass the damage that was done to you on to others. These actions might seem mysterious to you as they make you wonder how you could be so thoughtless and cruel to people you love.

When you catch yourself acting like that, don't punish yourself. It doesn't help to pile on more self-abuse. Instead, start wondering about your self. That's what Eckhart did.

That shift in focus might start you moving past your own personal hell. And it's a great first step toward bringing heaven down to earth.

To Decide

You have a choice: pass the trauma inflicted on you down to the next generation, your acquaintances, or your loved ones—or stop that process now.

Therapy can help. So can meditation. Those old traumas, and the pain associated with them, may bubble up under circumstances that allow you to let them go. You may not enjoy the process. You may even fight it. But bear in mind that what you resist, persists.

> Some of the greatest Learning Experiences are ones you'd never ask for.

I have to admit that, as horrible as it seems, that experience of hell within can be valuable in retrospect. I wonder if Eckhart would agree. Assuming you live through it, you may get to see what life is like on the other side of darkness. It's the proverbial hero's journey. You descend into darkness and confront the dragon. When (and if) you emerge victorious, you're different. You're transformed.

Some of the greatest Learning Experiences are ones you'd never ask for.

Why on earth would you request such suffering for yourself? Even if you don't, you get dragged through the knothole anyway.

Out of frustration, I once asked a therapist, "Have you ever met anyone who had great parenting, who had all their needs met?"

He thought for a minute before he replied. "Yes, I've known a couple of those people," he said. "They're genuinely happy. But they're not wise."

When you decide to confront your own demons, it's a momentous occasion. You've decided to embark on the healing journey. Remember, the word *decide* comes from the same root as homicide and suicide. Ultimate decisions kill off all other options.

Once you decide to confront the worst things in yourself, you may never go back. You've committed to healing.

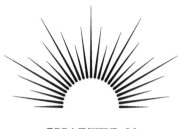

CHAPTER 20

Healing

Physicians go through years of training and practice to learn how to cure disease. Curing is a complex process requiring knowledge, technique, and experience.

Healing is different from curing. It doesn't require special training. Healing is not special. Anyone can do it. Some hairdressers and bartenders are really good at it.

Physicians can become good at it, to the degree that they decide to slow down and become aware of the I Am. And physicians are uniquely situated. Every working day they witness situations calling for healing.

Everybody needs healing. If you're alive on this planet, it doesn't matter how happy, successful, and satisfied you might feel. You need healing.

Why? Because when you die, you will let go of all those things that made you feel happy, successful, and satisfied.

Not coincidentally, when you arrive on your deathbed, you may be surprised to find that you feel unhappy, unsuccessful, and dissatisfied.

You may discover you didn't do what you might have done with your life. And you'll certainly discover that you can't take along any of those things with you that made you feel happy, successful, and satisfied.

There's only one thing you will take with you when you leave: the real *you*.

Ultimate Loneliness

Healing is the act of moving toward wholeness. It happens when you re-inhabit the I Am. It happens when you return, even for a moment, to who you really are. At that moment, you are privileged, just like I was when I met that baby.

> There's only one thing you will take with you when you leave: the real you.

Meditation is valuable because it quiets the mind, moving you out of your self and back toward who you really are—toward the I Am. So meditation is a form of self-healing.

Healing happens between people too. It's how I learned to *be* with people who are suffering. Healing happens automatically when two people meet together in the I Am. Not *their* I Am—*the* I Am.

The I Am is universal being, expressed in individual experience.

Being together in the I Am reestablishes the natural unity that is so easily lost when you are caught up in your self, relating to other people who are caught up in their own selves. That's separation. In other words, everyday life on this planet.

There's loneliness—that feeling everyone experiences when they're by themselves and wish they weren't. Some people can't bear to be alone, so they surround themselves with other people day and night.

Then there's ultimate loneliness—that estrangement you feel when you don't fit. You just don't belong. In its malignant, highly developed form, you don't feel you deserve to belong.

Or you're so far gone that you've given up on belonging. You're no longer a member of the human race. And you just don't care.

> The I Am is universal being, expressed in individual experience.

The only reliable way to heal ultimate loneliness is to re-member who you actually are, to rejoin the human race, to re-enlist as a member at a basic, sacred level.

No matter how low you've gone, you're still a functioning member, and once you've been there, you appreciate opportunities to help others re-member who they are.

Re-membering and Dis-covery

Your eyes are a portal to the eternal, via the I Am. When you're residing in the I Am and you look another person in the eye, it's an automatic invitation for them to join you there.

In everyday life in this world, where you take for granted that you are your self, looking another person in the eye is a take-it-or-leave it proposition. Some people recognize you and smile back, while others walk on.

When everything seems to be okay, caring is optional.

But when you're eye to eye with someone who's suffering, that recognition can be a matter of life or death. That suffering may have pulled that person out of the I Am into ultimate loneliness, when they need the I Am most—if they were ever aware of it in the first place.

Helping a suffering person return to the I Am through your own presence and connection is what healing is all about. It's helping someone else re-member who they are.

Healing is re-membering—overcoming the illusion that you're separate from others, or from the living universe.

It's also dis-covery—helping that other person uncover the commonalities of mutual I Am-ness. Healing is helping someone else re-member who they really are.

When you dis-cover the I Am, you're not realizing anything new. You're just unearthing that basic you-ness that was always there.

It's like coming in from the cold. Once you're inside sitting by the fire, it feels wonderful. And it feels natural.

When a person gets that *Hey, I already knew this* feeling, that's re-membering. It's dis-covering what you already know.

Love

The Bible talks about faith, hope, and love, and puts love at the top of the list. Other biblical translations mention faith, hope, and charity. Whatever you call it, love or charity, it's the same thing—giving of your own presence to someone else when they need it most.

That love is the simplest thing. Yet, it's the most powerful force in the universe.

Healers dedicate themselves to the proposition that dis-covery and re-membering don't have to be random events. They can happen through an act of clear intention.

When it comes to dis-covering and re-membering, nothing is random. Acts of love always have that alluring aura of inevitability. This feeling of inevitability leads people to say things like *There are no accidents* or to resonate with concepts like synchronicity.

When healing happens, it feels special. Well, in the ultimate sense it *is* special. It's an instance of eternity touching into this world.

Coming to know who you really are. Inhabiting that place in yourself. Helping others from that place. Summing all those things up and applying them is called healing. It's an act of love.

The Other End of Life
Ultimate loneliness often afflicts people who are dying. They've shed some or most of their defenses, so they're in a vulnerable place. Because they've lost a lot and are about to lose more, that vulnerability can feel like an open wound. But that vulnerability also makes connection easier.

When you're dying, many of the defenses the self locks in place in normal conversation are out of the way. So healing conversations can go to deep places quickly, without a lot of work. The work comes as you're preparing to be a healer. That earlier, preparatory work makes the important work, the work that really counts, a lot easier.

Death is the biggest challenge your self will ever face. You created, nurtured, and lived in your self throughout your whole life. How could it ever be easy to let go of everything you've developed so carefully for longer than you can remember?

Death may be sudden. That can be challenging for those who care about you because there's no time for them (or you) to prepare. Or death may be the culmination of a long process you go through as you adapt to chronic illness. Modern medicine has turned many diseases that used to kill suddenly into chronic illnesses. You now have an array of opportunities, unavailable until recently, to adapt and let go of those elements of your self that no longer serve you.

An integral part of that letting-go process is moving your awareness progressively toward the real you—the I Am. That's important if you're preparing to die or if you're someone who wants to learn how to be a healer.

Preparing for the end of life is all about letting go.

You can set your intent to fully inhabit the I Am. That's a useful thing to focus on because the I Am arrived here when you were born, before you became conscious enough to formulate any intent. And the I Am will depart from here when you die with you on board, but with the self you developed left behind.

You don't have to pack a thing. In fact, you may have some unpacking to do.

Preparing for the end of life is all about letting go.

When you die, the real *you* will review your life. You'll receive some great feedback. And what you'll feel best about are all those healing moments you've been involved in. Those times you were healed, and those times you helped others heal. In reality, they're the same thing.

There's no time like the present to start getting ready for that journey. And since there's no time *but* the present—now's the time.

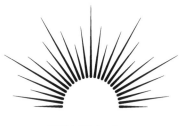

CHAPTER 21

Love

Physics tells us that everything we can see and know in the universe was created out of nothing. But even the vacuum of deep space, the location that comes closest to nothing—possessing zero matter or energy—still hums with latent possibilities.

Before anything existed, perhaps before the laws governing space and time existed, there was a total void. Yet (according to astrophysics) this emptiness still contained an incredibly large energy density that produced cosmic inflation, which in turn culminated in the big bang.

That was 13.8 billion years ago. But even as we speak, in deep space virtual particles are popping in and out of existence. Creation is, and has always been, happening everywhere.

If you're a physicist, you call it large energy density. The writers of the Old Testament called it God. For the sake of this discussion, let's call it Love.

Love is the energy that brings everything into existence. The energy that's so all-powerful that it continues to maintain the momentum of creation all the way through to the end of existence, when you leave. Or when the universe does, whichever comes first.

It's nice to call it love. That brings it down to earth and makes it useful. It also puts it into a relational context. Love is not just the force that starts everything in motion. It also attracts and brings nearby objects (and people) together. Without love, you couldn't imagine Hollywood or Paul McCartney.

Love brings us together physically, so babies can look us in the eye. Love unites good friends. I'm on a Zoom call every Saturday with the same folks I met in college more than half a century ago. The love is palpable—we often talk about it.

Love, Healing, and Sacrifice

Love also brings us together on another level, so that one person can help bring healing to another person who needs it. The intent to bring relief and a sense of peace and well-being to another person who is suffering always comes from a place of love.

You could call this kind of love *spiritual*. Christians refer to it as *agape*, the highest form of love and charity. It's the love of God for humans and humans for God.

This kind of love always entails giving away something valuable, some kind of sacrifice. Jesus's sacrificing his life was an extreme example. But when you're in a hurry, the sacrifice might simply be a moment of your time to stop and be present with someone who appreciates it more than you'll ever know. That moment of your time has ultimate value.

Healing involves giving away something ultimate.

When they say Jesus died for your sins, they mean he sacrificed his life so that humanity could find freedom. In Buddhism, the *boddhisattva* who has earned escape from the wheel of reincarnation forsakes it to remain in the world until every sentient being attains enlightenment.

When you engage in healing, you're giving your self away. Just for a moment, you're sacrificing the self you thought

> Healing involves giving away something ultimate.

you were. When you make that sacrifice, you experience the love emerging naturally out of the I Am in you as you connect with the I Am in another. There's no feeling quite like it—because it's ultimate.

That kind of love has one foot in this world. The other is in eternity.

Healing and the Self

When you engage in healing, you encounter causes of suffering that are of this world. At the end of life, suffering entails loss—of everything you know. The losses are of this world, whether they're material things, relationships, concerns about how others will manage when you're gone, or the ten thousand other aspects of life here.

Existential suffering and suicidal thoughts may feel like they're somehow ultimate. They may not map directly onto any specific aspect of life on Earth. But still, they revolve around a single thought: *I don't want to be here anymore.*

As Buddha said, "Life is suffering." But the suffering tends to come to a head when you're facing the end of your life.

When your intention is to help bring healing to someone who is suffering, that intention is triggered by the needs of another person, and those needs are related to the self. It's the self that suffers, and it's the self that needs healing. The I Am, the real you, doesn't need healing. It's the well you draw from. It's your source.

Deep Listening

You need to be careful of what you say to a person who's suffering. The impulse to fix the problem can lead you to say imprudent things, such as: "God never gives you anything you can't handle" or "Everything will come out fine in the end."

If you're suffering from death anxiety or major depression and someone says that sort of thing to you, it's worse than unhelpful. Those comments don't elicit the kind of energy you need when you're in dire emotional straits. They may just elicit guilt because you feel so far away from those good places, and it feels like your fault.

Those comments don't encourage anyone to take any constructive action. But it's worse than that. They may just make you want to kill the person who uttered them—or kill yourself.

The best way to make use of Love in the healing process is to start out by listening. Don't start by talking. If you start by talking, you're just trying to pacify yourself. Ask before you tell—if you need to tell at all.

We're talking about *deep listening*. You're not just listening to the other person's words. You're not just listening with your ears.

You're watching their eyes as you listen to their words. You're feeling with your heart for the presence of their heart. You're looking to connect with the deepest part of their suffering, and you're connecting from the part of yourself that has suffered.

That's why some of the best healers are wounded healers.

It's said that God makes the wound, God comes through the wound, God is the wound. I say *Amen*, brothers and sisters.

Connecting Self and I Am

When you engage in healing, you're engaged in a self-to-self interchange. It's their self that suffers, and it's your self that listens. But the interchange of love in the process of healing takes place simultaneously on another level. That level lies very close to this world, but it's not the same.

It exists between this world and the realm of the One Life.

For years, I had deep conversations in my medical office with patients who were suffering. They'd sit on the end of the exam table, and I'd sit on my wheeled stool below them. Often I had to let them know that their imaging studies and tests had revealed that their lives were coming to an end. Or we had already covered that, and now we were trying to come to terms with the consequences.

I say *we* and I mean it. Ultimate suffering is a lonely, isolated state. Far too many people are forced to go through it on their own. But if you're suffering and you realize that someone else is sitting right there in front of you, willing to *be* there with you, transformation happens.

But it's not only that you are doing something to transform *them*. Both of you will be transformed.

Humbleness

If you want to learn about that kind of deep transformation, you have to be willing to go down to the bottom—the bottom of your self. Over the years, I learned how to do that, in order to connect with others down at the bottom of our selves.

That's a deep place. No matter how difficult and uncomfortable the topic at hand, when you're there, there's comfort in just being together. We would talk, but eventually there would be no more to say.

Not because the causes of the suffering had changed at all. But because we got down to bedrock. The place where we both under-stood what was going on.

Then the time would come for the other person to get up and leave. On the way out, they would often say they were grateful. I would always say I was too—because healing is a two-way street.

You have to be humble enough to realize that you need healing just as much as anybody else.

Touching the Eternal

When you're down at that deep level, you're right in the middle of the I Am. You can feel it. It's the place where opposites come together. That's a big part of healing. Dilemmas resolve.

I became familiar with a feeling that, earlier in life, I would have found strange. Sitting with someone, dealing together with pain and loss, I would feel deep grief and great joy—all at the same time. They were blended in such a way, in that particular moment in time, that I couldn't tell them apart. Maybe in that deep place, they were the same.

At the end of the day, I'd go home and try to describe these encounters to my wife at that time. The conversation never varied. I'd start out enthusiastic, wanting to share what had happened. I'd say something like, "You wouldn't believe the talk I had with Mrs. Jones today."

My wife would say, "Sounds interesting. What happened?"

After a moment of thought, I'd say, "Damn, I can't remember."

I was younger back then. I couldn't use age as an excuse. It was frustrating.

Then I realized I couldn't remember because the conversation took place at such a deep level that the particulars stayed there. Then I would come back to the world and go home for dinner.

Maybe that deep level is connected somehow to wherever we go as we leave this life. Maybe, as we connected in a place between hope and hopelessness, we touched the edge of the eternal.

Maybe the love I felt for those people as I worked with them was connected to that ultimate love that creates and runs the universe. Maybe that's why those conversations were comforting to the people who needed to have them. And to me.

PART III

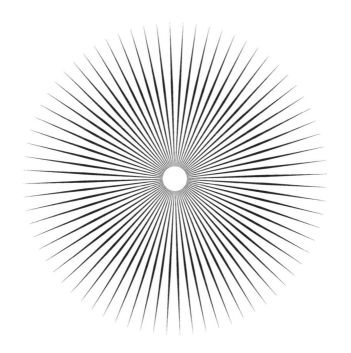

TRANSCENDENCE

CHAPTER 22

Meditation—At the Edge

Engaging in the act of meditation is precisely the same as placing your awareness directly in the I Am. When you meditate, you're there, sitting right at the portal to the eternal. It's so simple. And yet—it's not so easy.

Over the years, I've tried countless methods, books, teachers, you name it. I've been frustrated. I've been unable to make that voice inside shut up. For years at a time, I couldn't stay awake because I was sleep-deprived. I put meditation on the shelf for decades. Finally I just made it simple.

Meditation is the simplest thing you can do. It's the most straightforward way to be yourself—not your *self*, but the real *you*.

Meditation is also an extremely efficient way to surface issues that bug you, trap you, or hold you back. Then it provides you with a space to release them—to let them go, maybe for a minute, maybe forever.

That letting-go process is like cleaning house. As long as you live in your house, you are never finished cleaning it. There's always olive oil on the kitchen counter from last night's salad dressing. There's always a new cobweb up in the corner of the ceiling because that's the house spider's job.

Then again, there's those three boxes of junk in the basement from your last move, including those letters from that person you really want to let go of, but you can't quite bring yourself to throw them away. Meditation gives you a space where you don't have to do something as gross and disrespectful as throwing them in the trash. You just let them go.

Meditation is also the simplest way to sort out who you really are from who you think you are. It provides you a sword of discrimination—of the gentlest kind—to let you experience the I Am and your self, side by side. It's easy to tell the difference, and it's a vitally important distinction. It's the basis of real knowledge.

And finally, meditation takes you from Here to Nowhere. It takes you from Here, where your self lives in consecutive moments of your own creation, to Now-Here, where you live in the eternal presence of the I Am. It's empty, it's the void, it's the Source. It's Nowhere.

> In meditation, you're right past the edge of the world, suspended just inside the portal to the eternal.

This is not a void that intimidates you; it's the void that sustains you. It's good practice for when death calls and you leave here. The timing of that particular moment when you depart will not be up to you. The letting-go of your body may be a once-in-a-lifetime experience. But the real you, the place where your awareness will be centered, will be comfortably familiar. And if you put some practice in now, the letting-go of everything else will be somewhat more familiar too.

You may not lose your fear of death, or you may. Whether or not you do, at least the terrain will be familiar.

In meditation, you're right past the edge of the world, suspended just inside the portal to the eternal. In this space, you get to experience ultimate trust. Where you go from there is not up to you, but you know that wherever you go you'll be safe—far beyond safe.

The Process

There are so many instruction manuals for meditation that it can make you nuts. But the process is elementary.

You simply sit down or assume whatever position you prefer so that you're upright. Yes, you can lie down, but that can make it challenging to separate meditation from sleep—and they're different. When you're in deep meditation, you do feel like you're *gone*, but with experience, you can tell it's different from sleep.

It's nice to move your head around until it's balanced, so you don't need to use your neck muscles. You can close your eyelids all the way or partway, whatever makes it easy to focus inside.

In the beginning, there will be thoughts. Lots of thoughts. They are usually nonstop, and you may notice they skip around almost randomly, like gnats on a summer day.

You can try to quiet your thoughts, but trying is just another thought. Trying to stop your thoughts is like putting the palm of your hand against the end of a hose. There's lots of squirting.

Greeting Old Friends

You may find that old issues rise to the surface—things you'd forgotten about. Some of these might be issues you'd prefer not to remember. But there they will be.

You might try treating them like unexpected guests. Maybe you haven't seen them for a while, and maybe that is fine with you. After all, they were never your favorite acquaintances.

But don't be rude. Welcome them in, sit for a while. Then escort them to the door. You may never see them again, and that should be fine with you.

That's called letting go. The ideal place to be when you let those things go is right at home—sitting in the I Am. That's the only place where you can be empty of all the thoughts and feelings that make letting go such a challenge.

Kindly Discipline

There's a certain discipline to meditation, but it's the kindly type. Letting go to achieve your goal may seem contradictory, but it's a reality of spiritual practice.

Some might disagree. There are those who say you should meditate like your hair is on fire. They may reach their *goal* quickly. Hopefully, they'll achieve peace and healing eventually.

Others strive to control their heart rate, blood pressure, tolerance for cold or heat, or any number of other things that are normally controlled unconsciously by the autonomic nervous system. Some become quite adept at this, slowing their heart rate and metabolism down to the point where they appear close to death.

These feats of control (and others even more fantastic) are sometimes called *siddhas*. A whole science built around them has existed for ages in India, where they may be considered a mark of spiritual achievement.

Siddhas demonstrate that intentionally changing the activity patterns in your brain can have powerful effects on your physiology and your psychology. But awareness of the eternal may depend, not on purposefully changing the activity of your brain networks, but rather on turning their activity down—or even off.

Feel free to work on siddhas if you want. However, I'm not aware of anyone who has succeeded in preventing death, even though medicine tries awfully hard. That would be the ultimate siddha.

Meditating to Forgive

In the heat of everyday life, forgiving yourself can be a challenge. In meditation, that process of self-forgiveness can happen on its own. You may not try to do it, but at some point, you may notice it's happened without your knowledge.

That's a nice example of a benefit you might accrue when you stop trying and learn to let go. As G. K. Chesterton said, "Angels fly because they take themselves lightly."

You may discover that once you let your thoughts go and stop trying to control them, they start to quiet down on their own. They're like kids who used to rebel until you stopped trying to discipline them, and instead just sat down and paid attention to them.

You breathe in and out. You may choose to *return to the breath* because it's a calm, constant center of experience. You will always be breathing. It's a nice place to return to again and again. After a while, you're simply with your breath. The thoughts let up.

Paying Attention

After that, it's all about paying attention. First, pay attention to whatever is happening. A car goes by. The clock ticks. Then, relax into sensing whatever is happening around you.

That's mindfulness. It's satisfying, quiet, healing. You're getting there—but you're not there yet.

You may have a *mantra*, a phrase you repeat with each breath. That's nice, because it's another calm and constant wave that can carry you along, a wave you can return to. Mantras are sacred to some and ordinary to others. I've used many Sanskrit mantras. There's something mysteriously wonderful about Sanskrit. In fact, the word *mantra* comes from two Sanskrit words: *manas*, meaning mind, and *tra*, meaning tool.

> Enlightenment doesn't consist of shining the light of your mind into the emptiness of I Am. There's nothing there to see.

I think it's also fine to make up your own mantra. These days I just use "Aaah" on the inbreath and "Yaaa" on the outbreath because I like the sound of "Oh yeah," as in *yes, you're already there*. That tends to light things up.

You could try "I" on the inbreath and "Am" on the outbreath. But be careful. There's the I Am, and there's the thought of I Am. In this case, it's not the thought that counts.

So use whatever mantra you want, or no mantra at all. Just keep breathing and follow your breath. And invite your self to be quiet.

Turning Off the Light of Your Mind

Many people are confused about enlightenment. It's not a mental process. Enlightenment is not about understanding the eternal. Enlightenment doesn't consist of shining the light of your mind into the emptiness of I Am. There's nothing there to see. Enlightenment is about letting go of the light of your mind so you can experience the silence and darkness of your own pure consciousness. After you become comfortable with that, you may experience another kind of light.

Darkness gets a bad rap in our society. It's so easy to be afraid of the depths that tend to confront you in life, and especially in death. But you can't avoid those depths, no matter how hard you try. In meditation, you let go into those depths with intention, willingness, and trust. Developing that trust may help prepare you for the end of life.

Unfortunately, staying away from the edge of that abyss is programmed into you. That's why you and your physicians will conspire to do whatever it takes to avoid talking about dying—until you realize, through the process of healing, that it's safe to let go.

That's also why your self insists on getting in the way when your intention in meditation is to let go and penetrate the depths of your own being. Your self is trying to shine the light of your mind into the abyss of eternity. But it has no place there.

Turning off the light of your mind can be a useful move. If you're successful, your self may move out of the way and fall in behind you. That way, it stops being a headwind that holds you up. Instead, it may help you sail forward.

Don't worry if this takes a while. In this world, you have nothing but time.

Finding the Real You

Next comes the critical step, the step nobody may explain. The most important step in meditation.

You stop paying attention to anything. You stop paying. You no longer owe anything to anyone. Nothing in the universe expects anything from you anymore.

You let go. You become the attention. You are the awareness.

That's it.

It's like Dumbo letting go of the feather. You thought you needed to be mindful. Yes, in this world, you do need to do that. In this world, you need to learn to be present, becoming mindful of whoever you are, wherever you are. Perceiving whatever your self is perceiving, totally in this moment.

> You let go. You become the attention. You are the awareness.

But to move into the I Am, you must let that go. You must let everything go.

Then, you can move into silence, nothingness, the void.

Saying Goodbye to Your Self

When your self moves out of your line of sight, you may miss it at first. After all, it's been occupying your mind all your life. Once it stops doing that, you may feel like there's not much left.

Your brain has manufactured a self for you. Your parents and all your teachers have convinced you that you need to nurture and support your self. You have done your best. Maybe you have followed their guidance and obtained higher education. Maybe you have rebelled against their guidance and used lots of substances to dull your memories.

Whatever. You've made your choices. Now it's time to put all those decisions to rest, to leave them behind. You can reassure your self, and all your inner authorities, that it's just temporary. You'll be back to your chosen life in just a little while.

Tolerating Darkness

Letting go might make you nervous. Or you might feel bored. But bear in mind: you can't see the light until it gets dark.

Moving into the I Am is so simple, yet it's not easy. Once you're there, it's tricky. Because you'll immediately think, *Wow, I'm aware of being aware.*

And in that moment, you're aware of that thought that you're aware. You've popped out.

No worries. Just let go of that thought. Just breathe into the space behind your eyes and say "Ahh." Something might light up in your awareness. You're there. A bonus: it might clear your sinuses.

You might also notice a subtle kind of brightness appearing behind your eyes. Just breathe out and say "Yaah." Then repeat. It gets to be fun.

The Goal of Having No Goal

Finding the I Am gives you a goal, and it's positive. Striving to banish your thoughts from your awareness doesn't give you a goal to go for, and it's negative. So make your choice.

After a time, you may find that it's nice to have no goal. Your goal in meditation turns out to be nowhere. Or to put it another way, now-here. In meditation, you are now-here, so you are as present in the here and now as you can be.

That's the practice. Pure and simple. At first, you may find yourself doing nothing but repeating that process over and over. So be it. Ultimately, you have nothing better to do.

> In meditation, you are now-here, so you are as present in the here and now as you can be.

Meditation and Contemplation

After a while, you may notice that those empty periods grow longer, and they're very relaxing. You may also notice that time goes by quickly. Before you know it, if you open your eyes and peek, the clock says it's half an hour later.

You may notice that your thoughts don't always stop, but they change. They become simpler, clearer, and more useful. That confusing problem you were working on has a solution after all—and it's simpler than you thought. Because focused thought is not always the best way to solve problems.

You may even find that meditation periods are a good place and time to let some knotty problems untie themselves. But be aware. That's called *contemplation*. It's easy to conflate contemplation with meditation, but they're different. Contemplation is condensed, simplified, and flowing thought. It's another useful skill to cultivate in this world.

But meditation is nothing, nowhere, now-here. It's empty of *thought* content. That's absolutely useful, because it slides you right into the I Am, the real you.

Being in the I Am

Meditation is empty of thought content, but it may not be empty of *all* content. As you let go, you may feel yourself falling back. You may notice it's different from the familiar feeling of moving forward that you're used to while you're busy achieving things in life.

And you may notice that you fall back into a space that's, well, spacious. It can be a little disorienting. It's unfamiliar. It's not under your control. At first, you may feel like you want to get a grip, which is fine—go right ahead.

Then you may find yourself returning to that place. Once it gets familiar, you may notice that it's sort of warm and welcoming. It's kind of happy, in a calm way. Or after a while, it could even feel blissful. Or you might feel that you're being loved in a way that feels sustaining.

You can be like the redwoods when the fog comes in off the ocean at sunset. The redwoods can go without rain for months, just like you may go without healing and peace all day. Then the quiet of evening comes, and they just inhale the mist. That's what meditation is like.

Beyond that, we don't need to go. It's your choice whether to let go further into that space. You never know what you might find.

A Place to Come From

Some people view meditation as a form of escape. It may feel like you're getting away from your hectic life and going to a quiet place.

But meditation doesn't just give you a place to escape to. It gives you a place to *come from* after you return to your life.

Buddha didn't meditate to escape from the world. He sought and found the I Am because he wanted to find a solution to the problems of aging, pain, and suffering. Then he went out in the world and taught others that there was a place they could find in themselves, that they could come from, to manifest kindness and compassion in a world that needed those things.

Jesus went to be with the Father—the One Life, expressed in a patriarchal fashion—at night while his disciples slept. Then in the morning, he went out to preach the Kingdom of Heaven within to anyone who had ears to hear. The Kingdom of Heaven was where he went at night, and where he came from—both when he was born and when he was teaching and healing each day.

Buddha and Jesus were great healers. They brought peace on Earth because they knew where they were coming from. They also made it clear to anyone who would listen that they were just showing the way. Anyone can find that place to come from.

Back to Life

When you come back from meditation, from your journey to now-here, you may feel refreshed or calm. You may feel a sort of afterglow. Or you may not. You may just hop back into your life. But over time, you may find that you have a growing ability to simply experience each moment as you're in it, then let go of it as the next moment comes along.

That's what your mind was *actually* created to do: to let those moments flow, to let creation happen. Your mind may remember how to do that once you move back toward the ever-desireless.

When you're out in the world, that kind of presence may help you develop real mindfulness. The simplest things become profound. You may look up and say to yourself, *Hmm, that sky is seriously, extremely blue. Why haven't I noticed that before?*

Sometimes you might have an unaccountable feeling of gratitude. Or a quiet urge to rejoice. You may have sudden and unpredictable attacks of awe. You may be awestruck while you're viewing the universe on a dark night, or seeing a vast mountainscape, or hearing a powerful piece of music, or gaping at the intricate, velvety, crimson perfection of a rose.

Be forewarned—your political perspective may change without warning. The experience of awe automatically shrinks the self and its concerns, and instead stimulates concern for the world and all of humanity (van Elk 2019).

Social and environmental activism may result. Or who knows, you may choose to become a healer.

When you look inward with mindfulness to experience your own sensations, thoughts, and feelings—pleasant or unpleasant—that kind of presence has been called "restorative embodied self-awareness" (Fogel 2021). This awareness induces beneficial changes in your nervous system. It's very healing. Meditation is just the next step beyond.

These mindful things are what your awareness originally did before it got a little cluttered.

Meditation and the Default Mode Network (DMN)

In this and the following chapters, I'll try to describe some relevant, and perhaps surprising, scientific findings about brain function.

One of the most remarkable discoveries of neuroscience is the importance of learning how to turn certain parts of your brain off if you want to become aware of the ultimate and eternal. As with enlightenment, this kind of learning is the polar opposite of what most people have been taught that learning is all about.

This area of research is exploding. New findings and new theories are emerging quickly. I can promise you that at least half of what you read here will be wrong in a short time. I just can't tell you which half or how long it will take.

In order to express these complex issues in language, I'm grossly oversimplifying them. But a few references are included for those who want to take a deeper dive into the details.

When the brains of experienced meditators—those who have been meditating consistently for, say, ten years—are studied using fMRI, they appear to have undergone consistent changes in the brain circuit we've called the Default Mode Network (DMN).

The DMN was first noticed when researchers produced fMRI images of the brains of subjects engaged in certain tasks. Those tasks—in fact, any activity that involved paying attention—would light up certain brain areas. As we've discussed, this is the Task Positive Network (TPN).

Then fMRI was done on the same subjects at rest, so those scans could be used as controls. Researchers assumed that the control scans would show little or no brain activity at rest. Then the signals on the control scans could be subtracted from the signals on the active scans to get an accurate measurement of regional brain activity during that task.

But to their surprise, the rest scans showed activity in other specific brain areas, and that activity actually *diminished* while the subjects performed the tasks—just when paying attention caused *increased* activity in the TPN.

So they concluded that the resting brain defaulted to a specific kind of activity when nothing in particular was going on.

The term Default Mode Network (DMN) was born (Raichle 2015).

The TPN and the DMN work in opposition. When the TPN is engaged, the DMN disengages. When the task is done, the TPN relaxes and the DMN—the network of idle thoughts—comes back online.

The DMN is linked to creativity. It's active in dreaming during REM sleep. It's also involved in daydreaming, during which you may access REM sleep while you're awake.

Thanks to the Neanderthals

This has led to a fascinating theory linking modern human creativity to, of all people, the Neanderthals.

Humans spend a significantly greater portion of their sleep time in REM than do other primates. This may be related to our Neanderthal connection.

Neanderthal genes are found among about 2 percent of the modern human genome. Some Neanderthal genes code for narcolepsy, a condition that allows REM sleep to intrude into waking consciousness. This enhances neuroplasticity, visionary states, emotional learning, lucid dreaming, and the ability to connect widely separate ideas— thus creativity.

Science hasn't yet explained what caused the great leap in creativity that occurred from 50–75,000 years ago, catapulting us from eons of hunter-gatherer culture almost instantly into modern civilization. But that was the period when homo sapiens interacted (and interbred) with the Neanderthals, who had come out of Africa several hundred thousand years earlier.

It's intriguing to speculate that our current DMN—and our current hyperconnected culture—may have roots in Neanderthal genetics (McNamara 2021).

Turning your Self Off

When you're awake, your DMN is active whenever your mind is wandering, when you're lonely, when you're thinking about the past or the future, or when you're ruminating over regrets or failures. A wandering mind may be a root cause of unhappiness (Killingsworth and Gilbert 2008). The DMN is implicated in PTSD and depression (Nayda 2021).

This should all sound familiar. The DMN is associated with what we've been calling your *self*.

Your *self*, like most all things about you, results from a combination of your genetics and your developmental environment—nature and nurture. You were born with the DMN wired into your brain, a brain that has evolved to survive. As you grew up, you put your DMN to good use, developing a self that can respond to all the things that happen to you in your life, to refine your survival instincts in this complex and daunting modern world.

So it's not surprising when your self gets a little preachy.

This process of forming your self is, by definition, unconscious. Your DMN operates when your conscious attention is turned off. It's not really your fault if, as spiritual teacher Mickey Singer says, you have a roommate in your head and that person is a maniac (Singer 2007).

If you want to become free of this crazy cellmate before you die, meditation is one lead you could follow. Meditation has been shown to calm the DMN (Brewer 2011). The more experience you have with meditation, the better you become at quieting intrusive thoughts. You may find you get better at finding peace within yourself—just by taking a breath.

CHAPTER 23

Psychedelics—Through the Mirror

Psychedelics, used responsibly and with proper caution, would be for psychiatry what the microscope is for biology and medicine or what the telescope is for astronomy.
—Stanislav Grof, *LSD Psychotherapy*

A VW bus full of college friends and I were lying on the grass twenty miles outside of Philadelphia in Valley Forge State Park on that spring morning in 1968. When we arrived, we all took LSD.

There's a roaring. Maybe that's too strong a word. It's more like a potent, penetrating, subtle pressure, waxing and waning like a pulse of blood, halfway between a sound and a sensation. It's hard to tell where it's coming from.

I sit up and look around, smelling clover blossoms and crushed grass. There's nothing to see other than vast, green, sun-splashed fields, a few scattered granite monuments, and the edge of the deep forest behind us.

Maybe that sound arises from further away. Some factory? Probably not.

That roaring again. Maybe it's coming from somewhere inside me. I can't tell. It doesn't matter.

I lie back on the grass. The others have traipsed off in various directions. A solitary overstuffed white cloud floats lazily across the boundless sapphire sky, which is twisting subtly in intricate geometric patterns like it's alive. Maybe I'm watching the back of my own eyes?

A tiny black gnat pursues a leisurely zigzag course from left to right across my field of vision, just inches from my nose. He drones along with a robust, wheezy whirr, louder and more vigorous than his measly body should have been able to muster. There's a subtle aroma of overripe bananas.

I chuckle. My mind, playing tricks. That can't be a fruit fly, way out here?

I sit up and look back at the forest that takes up where the grass ends a hundred feet behind me. The trees surge with life. Their leaves are an implausibly deep and vibrant shade of green, extravagant even for spring. I can almost hear the sap running up from root to crown. The branches seem to undulate, even though there's no breeze.

I lie back down and gaze back up at the sky. Wow, that sun is bright.

This day feels perfect, almost unearthly so. I think about rolling to the side, but I discover I'm rooted. Long tendrils grow deep down into the soil from two spots in my upper back, just outside and above each of my shoulder blades. From a vantage point several yards out to the side, I can see my body lying on the grass, along with a crosssection of the ground below it. Those roots sprouting from my back look just like huge angel wings extending toward the center of the world, billowing as if they were immersed in a slow geological wind.

That's funny—when the hell did I ever earn angel wings?

Those roots dive deep, anchoring me to the spot. I don't mind. In fact, I'm overcome by the rightness of it. I'm filled with gladness. I'm one with the ground, drawing every drop of nourishment I'll ever need up through those roots. In that ground lies my heritage. It's issued me out onto the surface of the Earth, and someday, it will take my body back.

I watch that line of thought peter out and die. It gets thinner and thinner 'til it becomes translucent. I look through it.

I melt away.

As a human being with a body, I cease to exist. Or, more accurately, the unceasingly stupid, tiresome, overbearing perception that I am myself— abruptly evaporates. I feel natural, much more so than when I was the old me.

I nestle in a cocoon of sweet relief and release, vibrating with joy. But not in stillness. The heart of the universe pumps a torrent of juicy, wholesome gladness straight through me. That breathtaking cascade emanates from some ultimate and unknown source.

That's the roaring! An invisible, gargantuan, pulsating waterfall washes through me, fed by the mighty river of life.

That stream of bliss floods every inner thought and feeling, and every object in the universe, real or imagined, with ultimate goodness. Every single thing, regardless of how exalted or wretched each one might have seemed before, is now just glowingly right, perfectly appropriate, absolutely fitting.

Every thing stands exactly where it needs to be, and yet each is in constant motion and growth. And each is in perfect harmony with every other. At once, the universe is more than a collection of individually flawless things. It's a flourishing, superbly integrated whole.

All these perceptions are buoyed by a feeling of absolute, utter certainty. I have no doubt that this is reality, that I'm graced with seeing the veritable nature of the universe and of life. The ever-evolving universe of things is life, and the opposite is also true. Things don't exist. Everything taken together is a constantly changing, unutterably complex process, totally unguided but nevertheless perfect, free of any faults or defects. The universe is one huge, dynamic, unbounded, seamless, picture-perfect living organism. The absolute, the ultimate, pervades every atom through and through. It's all timeless. We're immersed in eternity.

Now, I'm dimly aware that time is passing. Thoughts appear like birds coming home to roost.

All things influence each other, nourish each other, depend on each other. Ultimately, they are each other.

Reality is indivisible. Our mind splits it into pieces. Our self wants to control it. But the second we do that, we stop the flow. We yearn to reach out and seize a fistful of reality, but before our nervous and greedy fingers can grasp it, it's already dead. Our crude intent to subdue it has already taken its life. We're just primeval hunters, killing our prey to consume it.

As we strangle reality in order to control it, we diminish ourselves. We abandon our own nature, abusing ourselves in the process. We become self-obsessed, willfully ignoring the magnificent truth that reality constantly murmurs all around us. We spawn fear and horror in place of the awe and wonderment that is our birthright.

We're born and we die. In our eyes, both entail blood and sorrow. But reality doesn't care. It just moves on without regard for our judgments. It grows, regresses, fades, revitalizes, flourishes, all without end. Maybe, in hundreds of billions of years, the reality we know will finally wink out, or disperse like dust in a cool breeze. But who's to say something else won't spring up in its place, or already has, inside other innumerable, infinitely varied universes we will never see or know?

I was back. I hadn't noticed. Sigh.

Each of us is so fragile, limited, and alone. From a cosmic standpoint, we're pitiful. And yet, each of us sits at the center of a universe of our own perception. And each of us possesses the capacity and the curiosity to approach all things, from the tiniest quantum to the ultimate reality of the entire universe, with love, respect, and even reverence.

That day I watched truth materialize right in front of my nose, as tangible as that fruity gnat. Then, as I fell back to earth, I wondered: *After I return to the distractions of normal life, will I maintain that truth or swat it away?*

Morning shaded into afternoon. Some of our group had paraded around singing all day, arms linked, imagining they were in a movie. But as the shadow of the forest lengthened, we gathered, sitting silently on the grass, leaning our backs against each other in a tight, outward-facing circle. The smoldering sun sank down sluggishly, like a warm red marble through honey, until it kissed the horizon.

We climbed into the blue van and drove back to the city, adrift on our own trackless memories.

Through the Looking Glass

Meditation takes you to the portal that lies at either end of life. Psychedelics show you what lies on the other side.

No one can know whether what you experience on LSD or psilocybin is *what it's like* after you die. But some aspects of the psychedelic experience are similar in character to near-death experiences.

According to research, there's now no question that psychedelics can help you accept your own death. The fear and depression that block many people from preparing for the end of life are lifted by psychedelics in most cases.

What you see during the peak of the psychedelic experience

> Psychedelics give you a pass through the looking glass.

helps you *get it*. Once you've been there, you realize that the separation you felt while you're living in your self is an illusion and that the ultimate and eternal unity of the One Life is the only reality.

Psychedelics allow your awareness to penetrate the mirror that surrounds your world—the mirror your brain creates to protect you.

Psychedelics give you a pass through the looking glass.

Psychedelic Medicine

A senior executive at a financial services firm noticed a nagging pain in his upper abdomen. Workup revealed that he had metastatic cancer of the pancreas. He declined surgery, as it would be debilitating but not curative. Chemotherapy was ineffective. His condition was terminal; his life expectancy was estimated in weeks to months.

Upon receiving this news, he became anxious and depressed. These symptoms worsened. Within a week, he had devolved from his highly functioning baseline state to one of disabling despair. He was unable to work. He stated that he was overwhelmed by dread and fear of annihilation. He was referred for psilocybin therapy.

After a preliminary meeting for psychometric evaluation and education about his treatment, he arrived at the center. He was escorted to a pleasantly furnished room where his therapist provided him with a blindfold, headphones playing relaxing music, and a measured dose of psilocybin. After he took it, he lay down on a comfortable couch.

He was quiet for about half an hour. Then his therapist noted various changes in his facial expression. About an hour into his session, he started laughing. Then he wept uncontrollably. The therapist placed a hand on his shoulder to make sure he was okay. He nodded, waved her off, and sobbed for a while longer. Then he lay quietly, not moving at all.

After a time, he sat up and removed the blindfold and headphones. Then he turned to the therapist. He still had tears in his eyes. "I get it," he said.

The therapist asked how he was feeling.

"I'm fine now," he said. "Thank you so much."

After a checkup, his wife took him home. A follow-up psychometric exam two days later showed that he had a fairly typical mystical experience. Measures of anxiety and depression were significantly improved over his pre-session testing. Those results persisted two months later, by which time he had lost twenty pounds and was much weaker.

He died several weeks after that, peacefully and comfortably, with no recurrence of anxiety or depression.

Psychedelics were studied intensively through the 1950s and '60s because of their striking psychological benefits. Passage of the Controlled Substances Act in 1970 put a stop to research, but there's been a resurgence over the last ten years (Nichols 2016).

To anyone used to working with terminal cancer patients (40 percent of whom have serious trouble with existential anxiety and/or depression), these results are game-changing.

One dose of psilocybin achieves far better results with severe cancer-related anxiety and depression (Ross 2016) than months of treatment with standard antidepressants or any other FDA-approved drug (Nichols 2017). About two-thirds of patients treated with psilocybin note improved mood and have significantly reduced anxiety and depression. Cancer patients also note that their sense of meaning in life is restored and thoughts of suicide are reduced (Ross 2021).

Patients with non-cancer-related depression who have not responded to standard antidepressants report that psilocybin changes their feelings of disconnection from themselves, others, and the world to feelings of connection, and also changes their avoidance of emotion to acceptance (Watts 2017). These feelings of disconnection and emotional avoidance are often worsened by antidepressant drugs and some kinds of talk therapy. A controlled study of patients with severe treatment-resistant depression showed that a single large dose of psilocybin reduced depressive symptoms (Goodwin 2022).

Humans have used both meditation and psychedelics in search of self-transcendence for thousands of years. These interventions each exert profound effects on consciousness, perception, and cognition, and they're synergistic when used together (Smigielski 2019). Meditation enhances psilocybin's positive effect, enhancing bliss, unity, and insight. At the same time, meditation limits any unpleasantness that might result from the ego dissolution that is central to the mystical experience that psilocybin induces (Griffiths 2018). Six months after newcomers start meditation, a psilocybin experience promotes feelings of interpersonal closeness, gratitude, life meaning and purpose, forgiveness, death transcendence, and daily spiritual experience compared to meditation alone.

Psychedelics also change attitudes and behaviors. Psilocybin tends to increase relatedness to nature and the environment, as well as altruism. It also reduces the attraction of authoritarianism. Whether or not this is a good thing shifts us into politics, which is beyond the scope of this book.

Psilocybin also works for obsessive-compulsive disorder, alcoholism, cigarette addiction, and certain inflammatory conditions. When they're given under supervision, psychedelics cause few side effects.

The Mystical Experience

Psychedelics reduce the fear of death by inducing a mystical experience. Without the mystical experience (for instance, if the dose is too small), there's little or no change in emotions, attitude, or behavior. The mystical experience has several components, and they can all be measured through psychometric testing (Barrett 2015).

The most potent (and clinically effective) aspect of the mystical experience is self-transcendence or, as we've been discussing, the movement of awareness beyond the worldly self and into the realm of the I Am, or primary consciousness.

Another term for this is ego dissolution. A 20 milligram dose of psilocybin is about equal to a 100 microgram dose of LSD. Either one will largely dissolve the ego in most individuals. Higher doses may induce greater ego dissolution but with the risk of more side effects (Holze 2022).

Once your awareness transcends the self, other elements of the mystical experience may unfold. You may lose your usual identity. You may feel you've been freed of the limits of your personal self, and you might realize you never perceived those limits while you were confined inside that prison.

You may experience pure Being and pure awareness as you see how restricted your awareness was when it was confined inside your mirror-encased world.

You may feel that you become absorbed into a larger—infinitely larger—whole. And because you have lost your self, you may realize that you and that Whole, that One Life, are one entity. Except entity is the wrong word, because entities are defined by their boundaries, and this Whole has none.

You may become aware that you are experiencing fundamental reality and know very clearly, without a doubt, that true reality is ultimate and eternal: Everything is alive and conscious, and nothing else exists. One is all and all is one; always has been, and always will be.

You may find yourself outside of history, where time doesn't exist. The whole concept of space-time may have been fascinating to your mind, but you've moved beyond that.

You have traveled from here to Now-here.

And yet—you may see your entire life like a movie with tremendous detail that flashes by in an instant. You may be struck dumb by some of the things you've done. You may feel the pain you've caused others because you were so unbearably unconscious—and then feel that pain as if it's happening within your own heart. It may be so excruciating you can't believe you could have been so cruel and thoughtless.

You may weep bitter tears at your own stupidity, tears from a well so deep it's bottomless. Those tears can cleanse you as you see the sense of what was done. You feel you can't forgive yourself, yet you're already forgiven because all your actions took place on a stage where the drama played out according to some unfathomable plan that makes perfect sense. Then you may weep tears of joy at the beauty and rightness of your life.

You may arrive at—or become—that paradoxical place where everything and nothing are the same. You become the void, where everything exists right now and yet also in potential, where creation and existence and destruction are all the same magnificent process. They come from emptiness; they are nothing, and to the void they will return.

And it's all exactly right—it's perfect.

You may have a strong conviction that nothing you're experiencing could ever be expressed in words. Language is so excruciatingly, pitifully inadequate to express the gorgeous perfection of the ultimate.

You may feel that what you're witnessing is so real, so true, that it's more real than the reality you thought was real before. This realization can be so vital, so crucial that you're convinced you'll remember it forever.

Underlying all this experience lies a feeling that everything, from the most delightful to the totally tragic, is ultimately and eternally good. You may feel the deepest grief and the greatest joy all wrapped into one. It's bliss. It's ecstatic and peaceful at the same time, and it's never-ending.

You may be consumed by a feeling of overwhelming gratitude just because you have the privilege of existing not *in,* but *as,* this blissful universe: You're in it, you're of it—and you *are* it.

You may feel the deepest, highest love for all things everywhere, past, present, and future. And it's not *your* love—it doesn't emanate from you toward some bunch of objects out there. This love *is* you, it's what you're made of, it's what everything is created from and sustained by.

Stephenie was right.

And because everything is composed of vibrant, living love, it's completely safe. You're constantly and for all time held in the embrace of that love, no matter what may happen.

You may come to experience ultimate trust because *every single thing that happens is perfectly right.*

All that taken together is why someone with terminal cancer who has been terrified of annihilation, once he's gone beyond himself and experienced ultimate reality, might finally relax.

Once he's laughed and cried himself through that experience, he might say, "I get it. I'm fine now. Thank you so much."

The Brain on Psychedelics

Just as the mystical experience can be measured by psychometric testing, the brain changes that accompany the mystical experience can be measured by fMRI. And like the psychedelic experience itself, the way the brain functions on psychedelics is paradoxical.

Psilocybin produces profound changes in consciousness. You'd expect brain activity to go off the charts. Yet it's the opposite: as the mystical experience hits its peak, only decreases in brain activity are seen on fMRI (Carhartt-Harris 2012). These decreases are maximal in key "brain hubs" that serve as connectors and integrators among networks that are thought to be associated with consciousness.

The brain hub whose activity psychedelics reduce the most is the Default Mode Network.

The DMN is not just a producer of daydreams, idle thoughts, and judgments. It appears to be the primary brain system associated with consciousness (Raichle 1998), the experience of the self (Gusnard 2001), and the ego (Carhartt-Harris 2010). The world-shattering experiences brought on by psilocybin or LSD result directly from turning this brain center off.

This is consistent with the "free-energy principle" (Friston 2010), the closest thing we have to a unified theory of brain function. It proposes that the brain constructs a model of the world that is very rough. It's just accurate enough to avoid whatever surprises the brain can predict. Only when something new and surprising happens does the brain put forth the work necessary to revise its world model.

Your brain doesn't create reality. It receives reality, and then strains out most of what it receives.

That model is always constrained. Your brain never shows you all of reality, just an estimate that's good enough so that—ideally—you survive.

Your brain doesn't create reality. It receives reality, and then strains out most of what it receives.

That's why you live in a hall of mirrors. You only see what your brain allows you to see. You can't see beyond the mirror. That is, until you turn off the part of your brain that does the constraining—the DMN, the part that constructs your self.

This supports Aldous Huxley's theory, proposed in *The Doors of Perception,* that the brain acts as a filter, letting through only that limited portion of reality that you need to go about your day-to-day life in this world (Huxley 2009). Huxley, who took LSD the day he died so he could experience his death fully, got the title of his book from William Blake, himself a mystic, who said:

If the doors of perception were cleansed, every thing would appear to man as it is, infinite.

Cleansing the doors of perception—cleaning the silver off your mirror—is a lifetime task.

But that's just preparation for what happens when your life ends. Then the doors truly open to what's beyond.

CHAPTER 24

Near-Death Experiences—Seeing RED

In Leslie Kean's book, *Surviving Death,* she shares the story of Pam, a thirty-five-year-old musician and mother of three young kids. Pam was diagnosed with a large aneurysm (a swelling in an artery that will burst if it isn't removed) at the base of her brain. Her prognosis was poor, and her only chance for survival was surgery. The procedure was high risk, but it was her only option.

The surgeon had to remove the top of her skull, then work his way around to the bottom of her brain to remove the aneurysm. Because the blood flowing through the artery was under pressure, he had to stop her circulation in order to decompress the aneurysm. This was the only way to remove it without risk of major bleeding. To accomplish this, Pam had to undergo hypothermic cardiac arrest.

After she was under general anesthesia, the cardiovascular team inserted a large tube into a major artery in her leg and another one into a major vein. The heart-lung machine lowered her body temperature to a target of 60.1 degrees Fahrenheit, almost 40 degrees below normal. At that temperature, her brain and the rest of her organs could be kept alive for up to an hour without any blood circulation as the colder temperature all but stopped her metabolism.

Then the surgical table was tilted head-up. Her blood was drained from her body, diverted through the machine. This dropped her blood pressure to zero, decompressing the aneurysm.

Pam's eyes were taped shut throughout surgery. Earbuds in both ears emitted loud clicks, triggering evoked potentials in her brain that were picked up by EEG. These signals are monitored continuously in all patients under deep anesthesia during this kind of brain surgery.

The cardiovascular team administered electroshock. Pam's heart stopped. It would not be restarted again until the surgery was complete—assuming it was successful.

During hypothermic cardiac arrest, Pam's EEG went flat. Her brain-evoked potentials disappeared completely. There was no blood pressure, no circulation.

All brain activity ceased. But Pam's consciousness did not.

She watched the surgeon over his shoulder as he removed her skull. He used a tiny rotary instrument that looked somewhat like an electric toothbrush. Pam had never seen one of these skull saws, but she described it later in great detail, even though her eyes were taped shut and the saw was packed away in an opaque sterile container prior to surgery.

As Pam exited her body, she experienced tremendous relief. Once she was out, she referred to her body as *the thing*. She felt it was beautiful that she was no longer a part of that thing. She was clear that she was *me* and not that thing.

She tried to communicate with people in the room. But although she could see them, they couldn't see her. She could move about the room at will just by thinking. She felt no more pain and no more anxiety, even for her children.

She sensed a presence behind her. She turned around and saw a pinpoint of light. She was drawn toward it. She felt a physical sensation as if she was being pulled by her tummy over a hill.

As she got closer, she discerned her grandmother and heard her calling, not with her vocal cords to Pam's ears but through some other kind of hearing. She saw many other people, some known and some unknown. They all seemed to be made of light.

She was certain she was connected with all of them. There was warmth and love, as if there had never been any separation. She felt she'd been brought there to be protected and prepared for something.

She encountered her uncle, who had died at thirty-nine. In life, he'd always had *the look*. He'd look at you and you'd understand. That's the way he communicated now. Soon Pam understood that everyone communicated that way, without words. She called it the *knowing*, because you just know.

She found communicating that way was much more efficient than speech. You just thought, the thought went out, and you received it like you were on the other end of a laser. There was no misunderstanding because everything that was said was the truth.

Pam asked her grandmother if the light was God. Her grandmother laughed and said no, the light is what happens when God breathes. That's how communication happens. Pam realized she was on some kind of light-filled bridge toward heaven, but they wouldn't let her into the source of the light.

Being a trained musician, Pam was fascinated by the sounds. Every being had their own individual tone. Many of the tones were very close together. On earth, that would be so dissonant that it would be hard to listen to. But when everyone sounded off in this place, it was completely harmonic, beautiful beyond any music composed on earth.

Pam came to understand that she couldn't stay. Her uncle escorted her back, which was okay with her. But when she saw her body, the thing, she couldn't stand the thought of returning to it. Her uncle told her all she had to do was jump, but she couldn't bring herself to do it.

She saw the doctors administer the first electroshock to restart her heart. It didn't work. Pam told her uncle no. She couldn't stand the thought of going back to that dead thing. So he pushed her.

She reentered her body just as the second shock restarted her heart. It was literally shocking, like jumping into ice water. She was alive—and very uncomfortable. It took Pam a long time to forgive her uncle for pushing her.

After she recovered from surgery, most of Pam's doctors smiled when she tried to tell them what she had experienced, but her neurosurgeon listened carefully to her story. He told her what she'd seen could not have been a hallucination. He consulted her medical records to confirm that they had had to shock her twice, which was unusual. That's apparently what happens when you hesitate at the brink.

Her surgeon was also impressed by Pam's detailed description of the skull saw she couldn't have seen. And being a musician with perfect pitch, Pam remembered that the saw emitted a D natural as it spun. When the tone of the saw was tested—but only when the neurosurgeon held it—sure enough, it emitted a D natural.

The experience changed Pam. She was no longer afraid of dying, although she still feared being left behind. She realized that grief is unavoidable in this world. But she envied people who were dying. She knew their journey would take them to a most wonderful place.

Science Travels Past the Edge of the World

Indigenous people have been using psychedelics to gain spiritual insight for eons. But mainline western culture only sat up and took notice in the '60s. The discovery and popularization of LSD jump-started a spiritual revolution.

Certain medical developments in the 1960s were just as significant—the development of resuscitation technology and intensive care. Prior to that time, victims of cardiac arrest were simply declared dead. But once it became clear that CPR could restart the heart, its procedures were standardized, and the practice became widespread. Today, it's common to see defibrillators on the wall in airports and other public places. As a consequence, millions of people who would have died prior to the advent of CPR have survived.

Near-death experiences, like psychedelic rites, have occurred throughout human history. But since the '60s, there has been an explosion in the number of people with interesting stories to tell after they were revived from unconsciousness following cardiac arrest.

Near-death experiences (NDEs) were documented and analyzed. Raymond Moody's *Life After Life*, first published in 1975, described the typical major characteristics of NDEs (Moody 1975). Still, even as reports about these narratives multiplied, their features seemed so divorced from the principles of materialistic reality that they were easy for scientific authorities to dismiss.

But so many survivors have told basically the same story that science has finally been forced to pay attention. Now experts from resuscitation science, the social sciences, neuroscience, psychiatry, psychology, emergency medicine, and critical care have published a landmark consensus statement and proposed standards for further research into what happens to human awareness after death (Parnia 2022).

Recalled Experiences of Death (RED)

Many related phenomena—like psychedelic experiences, ICU- or coma-related delusions or visions seen in states of religious ecstasy—have been lumped together under the rubric of NDEs. So authorities coined the term Recalled Experiences of Death (RED) to refer only to personal experiences that occur during potentially fatal situations, including cardiac arrest, that would cause the person to die without critical care intervention.

A RED is a specific experience that occurs during a period of unconsciousness caused by a life-threatening event. But the person undergoing a RED is only unconscious to an outside observer. People experiencing a RED are not just unaware of being unconscious; many report being in a state of awareness far more lucid than normal waking consciousness.

Raymond Moody identified eleven themes common to NDEs, as well as four others related to long-term impacts of the experience (Moody 1975). Today, about fifty themes are accepted as characteristic of a RED, along with multiple subthemes that have been added to Moody's original list.

These themes can all be organized into a series of six sequential elements of a narrative. It's possible that this series of events is experienced by all humans at the time of death, but only some can remember and report them later:

1. Perceived death and separation from the body

The person is aware they're leaving the body. The person knows the body was theirs, but they may no longer feel it's their body. They don't feel emotionally bonded to the body or to any of the activities in the room. They feel like a detached observer.

They feel they're rising up toward the ceiling of the room. They hover or float there without effort. From that vantage point, they observe the body and the activities of everyone in the room—and sometimes outside the room, where bodily vision can't penetrate. Their field of view is enlarged—they can see everything at once without focusing on it, as if they have 360-degree vision.

They know they're lucid, and in fact, their awareness may feel amplified, like a different and more comprehensive way of thinking and knowing. Yet they may feel confused or stunned as they try to figure out what's going on.

They come to understand they've died and cannot return to the body. They realize they've left others behind. Yet they feel light, physically and emotionally. They're both weightless and blissful. They have no cares or worries, no pain or problems.

They are certain they're alive even though they've been pulled out of the body. They know they still exist, just as they know the body is limp and lifeless. They realize they've shed the body like a coat and that the process was simple. It happened all by itself. They feel good to be free of it. Yet they witness a thin, luminescent silvery cord that still connects them to the body.

2. Heading to a destination

They become aware of a small bright light. They may see this point of light before or after they start moving toward it. They may not be certain if they're moving themselves toward the light, or if they're being pulled toward it.

Either way, they have a great desire to get there. They move fast, traversing a great distance. They perceive they're moving through a tunnel. It may seem dark, or it may appear to be composed of light.

3. Reliving an educational recording of life

They review a recording of their entire life—everything they thought, felt, and did. This review is like a movie running at incredible speed. Yet they see and understand every moment, reliving it as if they were there. It's not simply a review; it's a re-experiencing of each event in their life.

They feel the emotions involved in every moment, but it's not from their own personal perspective. It's from the perspective of those around them—those who were affected. As their whole life is relived, it's analyzed and judged with understanding and compassion, not condemnation. They see the good things they've done as well as the bad. They may realize they were not as good as they thought they were.

They are shown each time they had been selfish or cruel, choosing their own interests over the interests of others. They see every time they were divisive, every time they manipulated others for their own gain. They are shown every time they did something just to achieve an effect, and they feel how they actually felt at the time.

They see the domino effect of their actions, how they rippled through the lives of countless others. They see how their mistreatment of others may have injured those people deeply. They feel pain, shame, and embarrassment, sometimes quite intense, for those hurtful actions, or for the fact that they could have done so much more with their life. Yet these feelings are treated with gentle understanding.

They see how each of their loving acts also created ripples that spread widely. They understand how their seemingly small acts had impact on a large scale. They feel joyful applause for their selfless actions.

They realize that all thoughts, intentions, and actions matter.

Their life review reveals a natural law of cause and effect that seems almost mathematical. A lifetime's worth of particular thoughts and actions adds up to create a particular set of results, all making perfect sense.

> All thoughts, intentions, and actions matter.

They gain insights into themselves that they'd never experienced before. They realize they need to evolve into better human beings. They see that they are in charge of their own destiny, that something important is at stake—that they have a vital job to perform.

And they sense that this wasn't their first time here. They may wonder whether this was just one of many lives, each of which has a different purpose.

4. Certainty of being home again

The traveling seems to slow as they realize they are arriving *home*. Time has lost its meaning. Everything seems to happen in the present.

All worries, thoughts, opinions, and fears are gone. The place is pervaded by serenity and peace, along with a feeling of love, kindness, compassion, contentment, acceptance, and joy.

They meet a stream of other beings made of light, many of whom are deceased relatives who may look younger than they appeared before they died. These beings are there to act as helpers and guides, to answer questions and calm any confusion. No words are spoken. Everyone communicates by thought.

They may think briefly of family they've left behind. But they feel no sadness or regret. They're not upset or worried for them because they know they'll be taken care of.

They realize they're in the *knowledge place*. Their awareness expands moment by moment at a fantastic rate. Their knowledge grows exponentially— not about facts, but about the nature of reality. What they experience seems hyper-realistic. It makes their former life on earth seem like a dream in comparison.

The beings they meet emanate light of differing intensity. Some of these beings are made entirely of love. They are clearly superior in their knowledge of this place. Some are wiser than others—there is a hierarchy.

The person knows they are meeting the source, the spark of divine creation. They're returning to the origin of everything, and they feel unimaginable joy.

5. *Returning back to the body*

Finally, they reach a point of no return. They could potentially pass through, but they understand that if they did, they would be unable to return to this life. They are told that they're not allowed to pass through yet, so they must return to the body.

They want to stay because they are feeling more joy and contentment than the brightest moments life ever provided. But they're reminded that it is not their time yet, that they still have responsibilities. Despite their unwillingness, they know they must return.

Returning to the body is unpleasant. Some feel they are being sucked back in. Others feel their body bounce as they arrive. Some have trouble breathing and feel other symptoms associated with resuscitation.

They are left with a feeling of responsibility, a conviction that they need to fulfill their life's mission, to finish what they started.

6. Lasting effects after the experience

They feel the ineffability, the frustration of having to use inadequate bodily language to convey the majesty of what they experienced. They realize they've forgotten most of the flood of knowledge they received. They wonder if the brain and the body are even capable of holding that knowledge.

They use a wide range of different interpretations and imagery to try to describe what they experienced. They use concepts drawn from their own individual cultural, spiritual, and religious background and experience.

Despite realizing the errors they've made, they view the experience as extremely positive, perhaps the best they've had in this life.

They undergo a reappraisal of the hardships in their life. They feel their challenges were chosen purposefully to prepare them to evolve through their next lesson. They understand that they have a choice—it is up to them whether to accept those challenges.

They experience long-term positive effects. They become more aware of others' needs. They find it easier to put themselves in other people's shoes. They find it more natural to act out of compassion and kindness, although it still takes work.

They are aware that they still make mistakes. The experience has not made them perfect. It has just given them more of a choice about trying to be mindful.

Finally, they lose their fear of death because they've already experienced it.

In summary, a RED follows certain characteristic themes. It has an indelible, ineffable, and transcendent effect on the person who experiences it. It also leads to positive transformational change, reducing the fear of death and augmenting meaning and purpose in life.

The Brain and RED

It's possible that everyone who dies experiences a RED. But many don't remember some or all of the aspects of that experience.

Brain cells don't stop working immediately when blood circulation stops. A recent study described continuous encephalography (EEG) findings in an eighty-seven-year-old man with seizures after a fall resulted in a subdural hematoma requiring brain surgery. He had a cardiac arrest during the procedure. Although he was in the ICU, he didn't undergo CPR because, due to his severe decline, his family had signed a do-not-resuscitate order so he could die peacefully. Thus, continuous EEG recordings were obtained before, during, and after his death (Vicente 2022).

According to the neurosurgeon who published the study, specific brain wave patterns were seen just before and after the heart stopped beating. These oscillations are typical of those seen during memory retrieval.

"The brain may be playing a last recall of important life events just before we die, similar to the ones reported in near-death experiences," he speculates. "Although our loved ones have their eyes closed and are ready to leave us, their brains may be replaying some of the nicest moments they experienced in their lives" (Clark 2022).

We'll never know what the subject of that EEG study experienced because he wasn't brought back to life. All we know is that he appeared to have memory-like brain activity for a short period after his heart stopped. After that, he had no brain activity.

We also don't know what most people experience when they die and are subsequently resuscitated. They don't know either, because they can't remember.

Somewhere between 10 and 30 percent of people who experience cardiac arrest and successful resuscitation report a RED. That means 70 to 90 percent have no memory of any transcendent events. But that doesn't mean they didn't experience them.

When the heart stops, oxygen delivery to the brain stops as well—the same condition of *anoxia* that I purposely induced in the lab rats I studied before I went to medical school. If anoxia continues for more than a few minutes, damage to the neurons begins. This is the first phase of relative or *medical* neurological irreversibility.

Neuronal function continues during anoxia. Some parts of the brain can live for hours after cardiac arrest, possibly longer. There is a period of time, a gray zone, when CPR can reverse the dying process. But if the person is not resuscitated, all neurons die eventually, and this constitutes absolute or *cellular* irreversibility.

Depending on how long anoxia persists, resuscitation may not restore all brain function, even if it restores overall physiologic functioning as it reestablishes oxygen delivery to the brain. This is because restarting oxygen supply is a two-edged sword.

Paradoxically, reoxygenation damages brain cells that have been under anoxia for just a few minutes. It's ironic—unless oxygen is rapidly resupplied to the brain, death results. But it's oxygen itself that causes cellular damage when patients are resuscitated. Reoxygenation damage happens in other organs, too, particularly the heart (Früh 2021).

Brain areas associated with recent memories may be particularly sensitive to damage from anoxia, and when circulation is restored, those memories may be lost.

It's possible that everyone who dies has a RED. But not everyone remembers it.

Thus, CPR may have several different effects. If it's started soon enough, it restores circulation, and the body remains alive. It may also bring the person having the RED back into the body. It may also damage parts of the brain that remember the RED experience.

It's possible that everyone who dies has a RED. But not everyone remembers it.

CPR has allowed us to extend life. It's also helped us to study death. Without resuscitation technology and critical care, far fewer people would live to tell the RED story— assuming they remember it.

Science has unwittingly opened the door to exploration through the portal at the end of life. The view through that doorway is changing our conception of who we are and of what death is.

What effect could these new realizations have on science itself?

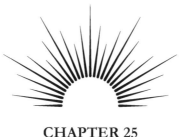

CHAPTER 25

A New Paradigm

Science is the best method humanity has developed to sort out what's actually happening in this world from what we think might be happening—or what we wish would be happening. Some say that's what the Enlightenment was about: moving us beyond the wishful thinking of religion to the objective reality of science.

But science has no authority outside the mirror that surrounds this world. It can't give us a real perspective—or any perspective at all—on the ultimate, the eternal.

Even inside the mirror, scientists can't reconcile the science of the cosmic universe with the science of the atomic universe. There is no unified picture of what we see at both edges of the self's reality—the deep universe beyond the self's outer edge and matter's fundamental building blocks inside the inner edge. So it's not surprising that science can't help us know what's beyond the portals at each end of this life.

The Hard Problem of Consciousness

Hi-tech imaging studies have given us increasingly detailed pictures of brain activity. They do that by measuring things like rates of glucose metabolism and changes in brain microcirculation patterns. When certain neural networks in the brain use more glucose or have increased arterial circulation (hence higher oxygen usage), they light up on imaging studies. When they light up, it means they're engaged.

From the point of view of human consciousness, what are those brain networks engaged in?

How do they produce the ten thousand things we see, feel, and think?

We have no idea.

We're starting to see how brain structure and activity relate to what people *report* they're seeing or thinking. But we don't know how the brain manufactures *what* they're seeing or thinking.

We have no idea how the brain produces consciousness. If it does—and that's a huge *If.* We'll examine why that's uncertain in a moment.

Imaging technology can show us patterns of brain activity, but it can't read minds.

What It's Like

So far at least, science has no way of telling us how the brain lets us experience seeing, doing, thinking, or feeling anything. This is a core dilemma in consciousness research. It's been called the "hard problem" of consciousness (Chalmers 2007).

The easy problems of consciousness (although it may take another century of research to fully figure them out) are things like reacting to stimuli, integrating information, focusing attention, and controlling behavior. All these abilities can be explained through garden-variety cognitive science using standard computational and neural models.

The hard problem is—what is *subjective experience*?

The wavelength of blue light from a clear sky measures about 400 nanometers. The red light reflected from a rose is longer—about 750 nanometers. The blue light emitted by very hot stars is red—shifted in proportion to their distance from us—because the more distant they are, the faster they're moving away from us and the more their light is stretched to longer wavelengths.

How fascinating. But how do you know what it's like to *see* a blue sky, or *smell* a red rose, or *wonder* about the expanding universe?

We have no idea. Only one consciousness knows *what that's like*—yours.

The Boundary of the Self

There is "something it's like" to be a conscious organism (Nagle 2007). That's the best current working definition of consciousness. If an organism is conscious, it's constantly experiencing *what it's like* to be itself. If you're that organism, you know exactly what it's like. It's like being you. That's your fundamental conscious experience. You know precisely what it's like to be your self.

But even if you're extremely empathic, you can never know what it's like to be another person. Making assumptions about another person's consciousness is risky business. If you want to know what it's like for another person to be who they are at that moment, you have to ask.

When another person is suffering and vulnerable and you ask them what they're going through, you don't stop and wonder if they're conscious. As a healer, you're trying to get as close as you can to what they're thinking and feeling. You're edging right up to *what it's like* to be going through what they're going through.

You're moving two consciousnesses together until they're as close as they can be. But still you can't *know* their experience. At least within the mirror around this world.

Science, Meet Mysticism

If there's anything to the hundreds, maybe thousands, of documented reports of near-death experiences, the evidence indicates that those individual boundaries may dissolve once you've gone through the portal at the end of this world. And if you have experience with meditation and/or psychedelics, you already know something about that portal and what may lie on the other side. You've used some of the available tools to get a glimpse. However, you won't *know* you know until you get there.

Science, under our current paradigm at least, ends at the portal. It also ends when it tries to explain your subjective experience. Science can't penetrate those boundaries.

That might change if we alter our current scientific paradigm. Mystics have talked about the unity of all things and the illusion of time and space for thousands of years. But mysticism has a bad name among scientists. The best science can do, even today, to explain consciousness is to postulate that the brain creates it—somehow.

Subject and Object

The Tao that can be told is not the eternal Tao.

The name that can be named is not the eternal name.

The nameless is the beginning of heaven and earth.

You can't name the eternal name because language is incapable of expressing the eternal. Subjects act on objects. That's the language of the self—the language of this world. And it's also the language of science.

Science assumes that the subject—an impartial observer—observes objects that possess their own unique properties. All the subject needs to do is measure those properties and bang—that's reality.

Two problems with that paradigm concern us here. There are more, but we'll stick with these.

The first problem concerns the dilemma that clinical medicine now faces regarding death. When you separate the subject from the object, you're left with scientific medicine that attacks the illness and forgets that a suffering person is involved. Once that rupture happens, it takes a lot of a particular kind of work to re-member the essential unity of life that makes compassion and empathy possible.

Until physicians and other clinicians learn how to do that work—and that learning hasn't yet been fully integrated into medical training and practice—healing will remain a lost art. Healers will have to continue to learn by the seat of their pants, making mistakes until they get it right.

The second problem concerns the nature of reality and of consciousness. Science today tries to make consciousness the object of scientific study. Our current scientific paradigm assumes that an impartial observer is doing the observing of the object called consciousness.

But consciousness is already the subject doing the studying. Even the most sophisticated scientific instruments observe and report absolutely nothing until their data are absorbed and interpreted by a conscious human. In the study of consciousness, the investigator looks through the microscope and sees—their own eye. Trying to understand consciousness this way is fruitless. The subject, the observer, *is* consciousness.

Science has discovered, as it investigates the behavior of photons, that it can't separate the subject, the impartial observer, from the object. Without the observer, there is no reality. The same goes for consciousness.

Studying consciousness as if it were an object is like trying to pick yourself up by your own hair.

That's why the hard problem of consciousness is so hard. Science can never tell me what it's like to be you.

> The primary reality might be consciousness.

Even if (or when) science develops machines that read thoughts, we're still trapped on this side of the mirror. Under its current materialistic paradigm, science can't answer the most intriguing question: Why does consciousness expand when the brain hub responsible for consciousness is deactivated?

Science must start considering the possibility that this world of matter and energy we're so busy measuring isn't primary reality.

Instead, the primary reality might be consciousness.

Materialism

This subject-object issue has only been around for a few hundred years. Many people blame science's shortcomings on René Descartes for separating the mind from the body, creating dualism that put space between investigators and the objects they're examining—between the subject and the object.

But the real culprit was Galileo. He's famous for disproving the theory that the Earth revolves around the sun. This put him at odds with the Catholic church, which was very satisfied with the old Ptolemaic theory that the Earth—and the humans living on it—were the center of the universe.

Galileo created the standards that today's science still follows. Before him, the first scientific investigators in the sixteenth century had based their theories on perceptual experience. Reality was about *qualities* their senses could perceive. Everything that shows up on the screen of human perception, after all, is qualitative. Consciousness itself is qualitative. It's old-fashioned analog, not digital.

But being a mathematician, Galileo decided to describe reality in terms of *quantities* that could be measured and manipulated through calculation. In fact, he specified that the only characteristics that material objects possess are essentially mathematical: size, shape, location, and motion. Everything else, all the qualitative emotional and aesthetic stuff that can't be measured, was thrown into the closet labeled "human soul" and ignored (Goff 2019).

No wonder the church didn't like Galileo. It wasn't just that he snatched the Earth and humanity out of the center of the universe. He also demoted the human soul to the role of a glorified wastebasket.

That was the birth of physics. The scientific paradigm, which defines reality exclusively in terms of what can be measured, extends from Galileo through Newton to Einstein and beyond.

That harsh approach has hit the humanities hard, but our world has reaped the benefits. All the complex technology that supports human life on this planet today sprang out of scientific, engineering, and industrial applications of that philosophy.

Because that's what it is—a philosophy. It just happens to be extremely practical. It's called *materialism*.

Materialism states that what's real is only what you can sense and measure. Nothing you can't sense or measure (or calculate based on some kind of measurement, like how science infers the existence of dark matter and energy) actually exists. As a corollary, materialism states that consciousness is nothing but a byproduct of neurochemical reactions within the brain.

You may be sitting there thinking that you know better than that—but don't be smug. If you're like most people raised in Western culture, you'll have to admit you accept that picture of reality yourself. You don't believe it? Wait until you get a cancer diagnosis. You will head straight to the cancer center, where materialism reigns supreme. If, heaven forbid, your treatment becomes ineffective, you will be forced to confront the limits of that philosophy.

Idealism

In the 1700s, Immanuel Kant was dissatisfied with Galileo's one-sided view of reality, so he developed the philosophy of *transcendental idealism*. He proposed that objects "out there" don't have their own independent properties. Those properties come from our own minds. Other philosophers like Hegel and Schopenauer developed these ideas further. Consciousness, they said, comes first. Then reality follows.

Unfortunately for idealism, the fruits of materialism piled up throughout the 1800s. By the twentieth century, especially in the very pragmatic United States, materialism ruled. Idealism was buried.

Then, in the early 1900s, along came quantum mechanics. Nonlocality, entanglement—even Einstein couldn't accept this kind of mystical "spooky action at a distance." But the measurements and the mathematics were airtight. Quantum mechanics is real and just as valid as General Relativity, even though the two don't reconcile.

Today, we apply quantum mechanics routinely in nuclear physics, astrophysics, and electronics. Quantum computing is about to revolutionize computer science.

What does that have to do with the nature of consciousness?

Consciousness Determines Reality

Quantum physics has been around for more than a century, but its implications are just now dawning on us.

Things do not exist on their own. They only exist in relation to other things.

In the physics lab, particles like photons don't seem to exist until you detect them. They lurk out there somehow in a haze of probabilities—called superposition—until your detector nails them down by making a measurement of one of their properties. Then, of course, an investigator has to observe the experimental results. Measuring those properties (and employing consciousness to do so) makes them real.

Nailing down physical properties is called *quantum collapse*. It's how reality is created. Physicists create particles of reality in their labs out of a haze of probabilities, and you do the same thing every moment of your life with your mind. Each of the moments you experience is an instance of quantum collapse.

> **Without consciousness, there can be no measurements.**

Galileo was only half right. He knew it was important to sort out that portion of reality that observers can measure. All the unmeasurables, including consciousness, were irrelevant, banished to the human soul. But what he left out—and science did too, until quantum mechanics came along—was critical.

Only conscious observers can perform measurements.

Without consciousness, there can be no measurements.

Relationships Are Reality

Quantum collapse doesn't just happen in the physics lab. It exists everywhere in large-scale reality. Things only get real when they interact with other things.

As far as you're concerned, the *thing* that does all your interacting, that brings all the *things* of your world into existence for you, is your own consciousness. That's *idealism* in action.

> **Reality is not what you think. What you think determines reality.**

You create your own reality by interacting with things. You don't realize that when you're not interacting with them, they're not there—because you're not there either. Your brain, which evolved to make you succeed in this world, only observes what you're attending to in the moment.

Today, this is no longer just philosophical speculation. It's in the math. It's relational quantum mechanics, championed by Carlo Rovelli (Rovelli 2021). Rovelli didn't intend to come up with a theory that challenged our everyday conceptions of what's real. When he realized what his and his colleagues' quantum calculations actually meant, he was stunned.

Reality is not what you think. What you think determines reality.

This is not about bending spoons or forecasting the future. It's more basic than that. Matter and energy, the entire universe of things we can see and measure—none of that stuff is primary.

Consciousness is primary.

Being Conscious

The I Am is your own individual consciousness. You can experience it once you help your mind, the voice of your self, to quiet down. The I Am is your own personal reflection of the consciousness that dreams the universe—the One Life.

When they say *As above, so below*, this is what they're talking about. When you're in the I Am, you're in harmony with the One Life.

But haha!—it's empty.

Be careful if you believe you know what's really going on. All you can know is what appears to be going on in your world. Ironically, you really must know what's going on in your world. You created it. And your self is experiencing it. So you should probably be conscious of it.

That doesn't mean you can control it. Because the One Life constantly and eternally creates it. It's out of your control.

The best you can do is to be as conscious as you can.

You might always want to do your best to be conscious. Because you will be judged—in a kindly way. But you will also judge yourself, and that judgment may be a little harsher. So doing your best in this life may be a good idea.

And that means being in the I Am. Then you'll be ready to be in relationship with someone else when they need it, and you'll be ready when you're called upon to leave.

But that's just what's good for you. Let's look at what's good for science.

Science and the Ever-Desiring

Relational quantum mechanics tells us two things. First: Because all things depend on their interactions with other things, this world is a closed system. This allows scientists to say that the fundamental laws of physics can explain everything that has ever emerged, or will ever emerge, in our universe.

But nothing exists in this world unless it interacts with something else in this world. Nothing exists for you in this world unless it interacts with your consciousness.

That's how you are conscious of the ten thousand things that make up your world. Okay, these days your world consists of more than ten thousand things. Your world is more complex than Laozi's world was, even if he was a librarian.

But here's where it becomes bittersweet. You're conscious of your ten thousand things through your ever-desiring self. Science is conscious of its ten thousand measurable things through its ever-desiring mindset.

Science was bred by our collective self to comprehend, predict, and control the things of this world. Talk about ever-desiring! But, as it's currently constituted, science can't become conscious about anything ultimate or eternal. Why does that matter?

Because only in relationship to the ultimate and eternal does your life have meaning.

The Only Meaning Is Ultimate Meaning

Religions, at least the Western Abrahamic ones like Judaism, Islam, and Christianity, grant two different kinds of meaning to their adherents. You matter *socially* because you're a member of your congregation. And you matter *cosmically* because God loves you—you're a member of the ultimate congregation (Prinzing 2021).

You can leave religion out of it if you want. Cross-cultural studies of near-death experiences show that an all-powerful and loving presence will greet you after you die. Individuals report their experiences with this Presence differently, depending on their religious beliefs. Individuals with no particular religious beliefs have the same experiences anyway—they just see beings made of light instead of angels.

Science is beginning to turn its attention toward these experiences, but it will take time for mainstream science to accept these findings. Mainstream science still operates under Galileo's materialistic paradigm. So, unless and until science steps up to a new paradigm that includes consciousness as fundamental to existence, its perspective will be limited.

> Only through the ever-desireless can you see the mystery.

Unless and until it develops a new paradigm, science will continue to be interesting and useful—but meaningless.

Only through the ever-desireless can you see the mystery.

Science will only see the mystery once it lets go of its willfully blind, single-minded devotion to the ever-desiring self and incorporates the ever-desireless, all-pervading consciousness of the One Life.

At one time, being human meant you were woven into the fabric of a *living* universe. All thoughts and acts were the product of, and were in harmony with, that larger Life. Whether the underlying intention was for good or for ill, all human activity had meaning—it was baked in.

It's been said that if all of human history were represented by a rope 100 feet long, our modern, scientifically based civilization would occupy less than the last inch. The rest of that rope represents the period during which humans saw themselves as part of a larger Life, the living Universe.

Come on, science, you're just a baby. You've only been around for the last 500 years of human intellectual evolution. That's just the last 2 centimeters of our whole 100 yards.

Our Conscious Universe

Matter doesn't actually exist. Matter is how our brains perceive and interpret universal consciousness.

> Matter is how our brains perceive and interpret universal consciousness.

Philosopher and computer engineer Bernardo Kastrup's *analytic idealism* states that the universe exists in your mind, but not just your mind alone. The universe may be an intricately interwoven complex of quantum energy fields, but that definition is at the level of present-day physics.

At the level of the ultimate and eternal—and tomorrow's science—the universe is a transpersonal field of mentation—consciousness—that presents itself to each of us as the physical world (Kastrup 2019). We're all perceiving the same consciousness, so we all see basically the same universe. Yet, while you're here in this world, you perceive this consciousness through your own personal transceiver—your brain.

Is it true that no (hu)man is an island? Yes and no. Your brain creates your self, which is separate from all other selves, but you're partaking of the same unified field of consciousness as everyone else. And not just every other human. You and your dog. You and your cat, assuming your cat is in the mood.

Me and you and the redwoods. Us and the mountains, including all the *living* rock they're composed of. Everything is alive because everything emerges from that universal consciousness—while you observe it.

All this doesn't mean that the world is just your own personal hallucination or an act of your imagination. What quantum mechanics is telling us is that all matter is the outer expression of your—and everyone else's—inner experience. Various unique appearances of matter just reflect different modes of mental activity (Kastrup 2018).

It's time for science to advance past Galileo's quantitative materialism and bring qualitative experience—consciousness—back into the equation.

CHAPTER 26

Transformation

Humans, having developed the capacity to remember the past and imagine the future, are tortured by the awareness that they, and everything they know and love, are inevitably subject to annihilation.

The fear of death is universal. Everybody has it, and everybody represses it. If you didn't repress it, you couldn't function in this world. Most of the belief systems and institutions humans have created were brought into being for the express (but unconscious) purpose of keeping us firmly embedded in our denial of death. It's been said that this is the *why* of human existence. Ernest Becker won the Pulitzer Prize in 1974 for pointing this out in a comprehensive and artful way (Becker 2007).

Realizing that you are going to die—really getting it, down to the marrow of your bones—is unbearable. You'll do anything to pull off some kind of mental trickery that convinces you you're immortal, so you aren't forced to remember the fact that you're not.

You see this drama play out every day in every hospital in the Western world. Patients and their doctors conspire to pretend that everything is under control even when death is clearly approaching. You'll do whatever it takes to get better—or to pretend you'll get better, regardless of evidence to the contrary—because the alternative to that delusion is too terrible to contemplate.

And that alternative is: You know you'll lose everything, then you'll cease to exist.

No One Is Immune

Some people approach death without fear and instead approach it with calmness and equanimity. Sometimes it's the people you'd least expect— criminals, psychopaths, and fools. In ancient times (and perhaps now, although the term is out of fashion), it was saints.

Meanwhile, well-meaning, clear-thinking people today delude themselves into believing they don't need to prepare themselves to die. It's not that they're wrong or crazy. It's just that while you're living on this planet centered in your self, you can easily be fooled into thinking that you have the fear of dying under control.

Then when you're faced with death—surprise. You don't have it wired after all.

Even with a lot of practice, when you're facing death, you may have to work hard to get back to who you really are—the I Am. Or you may benefit from a little assistance from your local healers.

One of my hospice teams once cared for a close personal associate of the Dalai Lama, who happened to be visiting our area. This member of his entourage suddenly suffered some acute complaints. He was diagnosed with cancer and was seen at a leading comprehensive cancer center near us. He underwent the most advanced cancer treatment in the world, but it didn't help.

If anybody should have been able to handle impending death with equanimity, you'd have thought it would be him. Not so. He grabbed at every medical straw he was offered. He was terrified. Not because he had somehow failed at his spiritual practice. But because, like you, he was human.

And because he was human, he could only know how overwhelming his fear of death would turn out to be once he was forced to face it. All his efforts to understand death prior to that, no matter how spiritual, took place in his imagination.

He was too ill to be transported home. After several refusals, he finally consented to hospice. Our hospice team saw him at his hotel. Our chaplain was honored to meet him. Everyone—the nurses, social workers, therapists—had deep conversations with him. Lots of learning took place by all parties concerned. He died peacefully.

Be careful with your beliefs. All we know about what happens after death comes from the RED experiences of people who have not really died. You may say you believe that after you die, your soul will go to heaven. Or that you'll be reincarnated so you don't really have to worry about death. Or whatnot.

Whoever tells you they know what *really* happens after death is giving you a sales pitch.

They want you to buy their beliefs. Those beliefs may enable you to put off dealing with your own demise. You'll do that at first—until you receive a terminal diagnosis. Then comes the letting-go process, otherwise known as healing.

Through the Mirror

So many things can trap you in this world, making the mirror that encases it seem more and more opaque. If you're one of those people that follows the news, you may feel like the ten thousand things perceived by the ever-desiring mind are multiplying too fast for us manage them. And 9,999 of those things might consist of stuff you'd rather avoid.

You can't begin to list all the maladies in the world because new ones spring up before you can comprehend the old ones. Wars we thought were outmoded spring up in our own backyard. Foreign aid that used to be measured in dollars is now dominated by weapons systems. Viruses we never knew existed cause pandemics that kill millions, shut down our way of life, and disable our healthcare systems. Climate change fosters wildfires, tornadoes, and floods, threatening the existence of our communities.

Suddenly everyone is talking about *existential threats*.

A generation ago, it seemed like everyone believed in progress. Now being progressive places the believer in a warring camp. Tribalism splits us into warring camps that communicate only through hate speech that just echoes through the camp where it originated.

How entertaining.

Domestic spiritual wars seem especially demoralizing. Fundamentalism afflicts right-wing religious groups. Members of the very same denominations that used to preach love and tolerance now promote gun rights. But fundamentalism also plagues secular humanists who espouse atheism, principles of free inquiry, ethics based upon reason, and a commitment to science and democracy—and who attack the religious, comparing "those who believe that god favors thuggish, tribal human designs, and *those who don't believe in god and who oppose thuggery and tribalism on principle*" (Flynn 2002). That rhetoric is not intended to bridge the divide.

Maybe you don't watch the news or follow science. Maybe you're into entertainment. Just watch the Academy Awards and tally up the number of Oscars that go to movies with a positive, uplifting message. Then count the number that go to films that glorify criminals and psychopaths. You already know which category will wind up on top.

Politics today? That's beyond the scope of this discussion. Twenty years from now, either we'll wonder how people could ever have been as crazy as we are today—or what we consider crazy now will look tame by then. However it goes—it's the way of the world.

Science and Despair

Science is a two-edged sword. Every week, we announce new ways to cure terrible diseases. But science is powerless to heal.

Science is value-free. That's natural and necessary. Values introduce bias by their very nature. Scientific studies must remain objective and free of bias, so values have no place there.

However, when values are banished, the remaining world can feel pretty bleak. Nobel-prize-winning theoretical physicist Steven Weinberg writes, "The more the universe seems comprehensible, the more it seems pointless" (Weinberg 1977).

As a devotee of science myself, it's painful to say this. Science divorced from spirit has bound our shining city on a hill in chains of despair.

Here's a brief factual summary of the current status of the human race from a strictly scientific viewpoint: Humans are the product of a random process that has no cause. All our loves, hopes, and fears are the result of chance combinations of organic molecules. No individual act of heroic imagination, valiant action, or inspired striving will last beyond the grave, except for the fading memories of survivors who won't last long themselves. All the products of human genius are destined to vanish in the frigid death of an expanding universe.

How uplifting.

When the Enlightenment took spirituality out of the picture just five hundred years ago, the bottom dropped out of meaning. This disenchanted void is the emptiness of the present-day self. It's the exact opposite of the eternally creative void that characterizes the I Am—the gateway to ultimate meaning.

Mysticism in Plain Sight

Meanwhile, behind and underneath this bleak scene, another narrative is unfolding. More people have experienced meditation, psychedelics, and near-death experiences than ever before.

In 2012, the number of meditators in the U.S. was 13 million. In 2017, according to the U.S. Centers for Disease Control and Prevention, over 46 million people practiced meditation. Over those five years, meditation grew by 250 percent. In 2022, the Pew Research Center reported that 40 percent of the U.S. population—about 133 million people—meditate at least once a week (Pew Research Center 2022). That's ten times more than ten years ago.

It's estimated that, as of ten years ago, over 30 million people in the U.S. had tried psychedelics (Krebs 2013). Studies show that under the right kind of supervision, psychedelics yield life-changing, transformational insights and reduce the fear of death—and these effects persist long after the peak experience is over.

Thanks to the development of resuscitation techniques and intensive care, uncounted millions of people have died from cardiac arrest, had their hearts restarted, and lived to talk about their remembered experiences of death, a.k.a. near-death experiences. Almost all experiencers report that their fear of death was eliminated, often permanently.

You'll notice that a lot of people have been having mystical or transcendental experiences lately. Mystics are no longer just loners forsaking society to fast in the desert or live in a cave. We are everywhere.

Once a large enough number of people in any group—including a whole nation—have experiences that change their beliefs, the entire group's beliefs will eventually change in that direction. This never happens all at once. First, it's the early adopters. They're on the initial, gradually upsloping left-hand tail of the curve. The curve slopes upward more and more until it hits a tipping point. Then it goes nearly vertical as a rapidly growing number of people absorb the message. That may be where our society lies on this curve today.

You won't know by observing the media. The old newspaper adage still rules, whether it's print, cable, or online: *if it bleeds, it leads*. You'll only find those heartwarming little stories about young hospice volunteers sitting with elderly dying patients at the tail end of the newscast after the fifth commercial break—if you ever see them at all.

> A spiritual transformation of our society may be well underway.

Spiritual awakening won't make the headlines anytime soon, short of some freaky mass levitation event that may have nothing to do with finding out who you really are anyway. But still.

A spiritual transformation of our society may be well underway.

The Consciousness Question
After a lifetime of experience on this planet, you assume you know who you are. But consider the evidence:

You meditate. You find yourself in a deep stillness. The more you let go, the more you feel enveloped in a safe and loving presence. You're right inside the I Am, the portal between your world and the One Life. You can feel the Source.

You take psilocybin. Suddenly you're through the portal. You see how reality is actually constructed. It makes complete sense. You have incurable cancer, and you were in mortal terror of dying—but not anymore. You've traveled through that fear and out the other side. *I get it. I'm fine. Thank you so much.*

Your heart stops. You leave your body and travel to realms so overwhelmingly joyous and loving that you couldn't have imagined them while you were alive. You don't want to return, but you do. It's not your time yet, but you no longer dread the time when you will eventually, inevitably, die. You appreciate the life you're back to living more than you did before. Yet you envy those who have already departed on their journey, who have left for good through the portal on the far end of life—because you know where they're going.

Meanwhile, today *your self* is sitting here reading this. Your self—that person you believe you've always been. You're more familiar with your self than you are with your favorite pair of jeans.

Take notice. You're conscious. As you read this, you may become conscious of being conscious. It's a miracle. Yet to you, it's the simplest thing.

It's the most basic, fundamental fact of your existence. It's also a complete mystery.

We've talked about science and consciousness. Now let's talk about you.

Less Brain, More Consciousness

If you've thought about it at all, you probably buy the current materialistic theory that your brain, that magnificently hyperconnected piece of wet machinery inside your skull, the most complex object in the known universe, constructs your consciousness from the ground up.

That theory holds that your brain's billions of neurons, networked through trillions of synapses and other kinds of intercellular connectors, produces the experience of what it's like to be hit by an apple falling on your head, what it's like to get carried away by a piece of great art or music, what's like to fall in love. And what it's like to be you.

If that theory is true, then why do certain experiences—associated with meditation, psychedelics, and RED, each one more sacred and sublime than the last—happen only when the functioning of your brain is turned down, step by step—until finally it's turned off completely?

If those higher states of consciousness were produced by your brain like science assumes, you'd expect your fMRI on meditation to light up like a Christmas tree, on psilocybin to blast off like a fireworks display, in a RED experience to erupt like the New Year's stroke of midnight in Times Square.

Yet it's the opposite. In meditation, your Default Mode Network, the brain hub that's associated with your sense of self, is turned down. With a high enough dose of psychedelics, your DMN gets disconnected—the plug is pulled—from your self. In a RED experience, your brain shuts down completely—no detectable activity at all. You only remember it—if you're lucky enough to remember anything—after your brain is restarted. And while your brain is completely inactivated and your eyes are taped shut, you see things like skull saws and your own CPR that your eyes couldn't possibly have witnessed.

How unscientific.

Disabling the Self to See Reality

Maybe these phenomena are not unscientific at all. Where mysticism is concerned, maybe science needs to wake up to the reality that its own imaging technology reveals.

We've long suspected that many of the great spiritual and religious visionaries throughout history had their world-changing visions while they were in altered states of consciousness. And their consciousness may have been altered by conditions that temporarily disabled parts of their brains.

Neurologist Michael Trimble points out that many religious visions that have literally altered human history may have occurred while visionaries were having a certain type of epilepsy called (among other clinical terms) *partial complex seizures*. Saint Paul's conversion on the road to Damascus was accompanied by three days of blindness and episodes of falling to the ground. Muhammed described his own auditory and visual hallucinations during falling spells. Joseph Smith, the founder of Mormonism, reported periods of unconsciousness and an inability to speak, after which he woke up lying on his back and staring up at heaven (Trimble 2008).

People who aren't afflicted (or blessed) with this type of epilepsy now have increasing access to substances that can produce the same visionary effects without having to endure the physical disabilities.

Other brain insults can also induce mystical visions. Jill Bolte Taylor, herself a highly-trained research neuroscientist, describes her own sensations and thoughts while she was in the midst of a major stroke due to the rupture of an undiagnosed blood vessel malformation within the left side of her brain—the location of one of the principal centers that mediate what we're calling *the self*.

As her self shut down, spiritual overtones emerged:

As the language centers in my left hemisphere grew increasingly silent and I became detached from the memories of my life, I was comforted by an expanding sense of grace. In this void of higher cognition and details pertaining to my normal life, my consciousness soared into an all-knowingness, a "being at one" with the universe, if you will. In a compelling sort of way, it felt like the good road home, and I liked it (Taylor, 2009).

A materialistic scientist might see this report as evidence that spiritual awareness, the consciousness of eternal reality, always exists in the right hemisphere of the brain and it's just unmasked when the left side of the brain is inactivated.

Maybe that's true. Meditation might calm the left brain, shutting down the source of self-talk that chatters incessantly to keep you locked into *reality*. But still, why do psychedelics and RED experiences, which affect both sides of the brain equally, expand consciousness so dramatically?

> Maybe the entire universe is conscious, and your own personal awareness is a doorway.

The Brain: Receiver and Filter

Perhaps something else is going on. Maybe Aldous Huxley was right. Your brain isn't a creator of consciousness—it's a receiver. Maybe the entire universe is conscious, and your own personal awareness is a doorway. Or maybe your brain is like a cellphone, picking up universal signals and translating them into pixels on the screen of your mind.

Maybe the great majority of that larger consciousness, most of which has nothing to do with your bodily survival, doesn't ever make it through to your awareness—unless the filter is partially disabled by meditation or psychedelics, or taken down totally by death.

Maybe, if you perceived the whole spectrum of the universe's consciousness, just for the briefest moment, it would be like standing too close to the sun. Your survival would be over. From the perspective of your life on this planet, that filter may be a lifesaver.

That receiver/filter concept isn't so far-fetched. For most of human history, we assumed that visible light was all there was to see. Now our instruments tell us that the light the human eye perceives is just a small portion of the full spectrum of electromagnetic radiation that extends from the lowest-frequency radio waves to the highest-frequency cosmic rays.

We know that many of our own physical and mental processes are normally suppressed out of awareness. You can demonstrate that to yourself in meditation. Normally, you don't hear your heartbeat or feel your pulse internally. But once the jabber of your mind quiets down, you can perceive those things and many other bodily processes that are normally outside of awareness—if you choose to. Try staring at a white wall. If you're patient, you'll see the red blood cells flowing through the capillaries in your retina.

A Spectrum of Consciousness

Likewise, you repressed those hurtful memories and thoughts, those products of the abuse and neglect many of us suffered when we were too young to defend ourselves. You pushed those indecent memories into your unconscious so you could go about your life without the constant pain you'd feel if they intruded into your awareness.

Well, they manifest anyway in the neuroses, phobias, and substance abuse that may bug you, but those annoyances are manageable as long as they don't disable you. That's why neuroses are called defense mechanisms. They defend you against the things you don't want to be aware of. Being neurotic is easier on you than reliving those obnoxious memories.

In meditation, those old friends can be de-repressed, sometimes accompanied by the pain that was stored alongside. That's why staying centered in the I Am is so useful. While you're in that place, you can greet those old acquaintances calmly without getting sucked into the vortex of their presence—and then show them the door. That's the letting-go process in action.

By the way, I am *not* recommending you substitute meditation for psychotherapy. But it's a nice adjunct, and it's a lot cheaper.

What if there's a spectrum of internal consciousness that's different from, but analogous to, the electromagnetic spectrum? All that repressed unconscious material may correspond to the low-frequency infrared part of the spectrum. Sitting above that might be your everyday awareness, like visible light. Then above the upper edge of your awareness, there may lie a vast region of higher-frequency awareness-in-potential beyond the ultraviolet.

You might experience various ranges of those higher-energy frequencies differently depending on the particular consciousness-modifier you choose to employ. The list includes meditation, psychedelics, near-death experiences (you may not want to try that one at home), or countless others, such as breathwork or simply taking a hike in the mountains. You'd experience each of those differently, just as you perceive TV, radio, and heating up leftovers in the microwave as different even though they all function on the same range of wavelengths.

It's exciting to contemplate the possibility that once science grows into accepting consciousness as primary reality, we might discover that what we now regard as the unconscious might become accessible to human awareness. That might cast a new light on the nature of time, distance, and other parameters of present-day *reality* that we now regard as immutable.

Your Little Spark

Consciousness may be some kind of emanation. We just don't know what kind. That's okay—we don't know what kind of emanation gravity is either, but we're on track to find out. We also don't know what dark matter or dark energy are. All we know is that, taken together, they make up 95 percent of the matter/energy content of the universe. The normal matter we can perceive (and that everything we know is composed of) only comprises 5 percent of the total.

No one can know this for sure—except maybe certain mysterious sages in the East—but that 5 percent figure might match the minute proportion of universal consciousness you can be aware of while you're living a normal life in your body. You might be able to expand your range if you're diligent or lucky.

Maybe science's current materialistic paradigm has it wrong. Maybe the brain doesn't create consciousness. Maybe consciousness is the fundamental substance of the universe. Maybe our little individual consciousnesses are just damped-down manifestations, tiny sparks, of universal consciousness.

That's what mystics have been saying throughout history and before history was recorded. And that awakening may be coming soon to a brain near you—the one inside your very own skull.

Awakening

Our whole society, our entire culture, the entire world, is waking up. Heaven is coming down to earth. You, everyone you know or encounter— all of us—are collaborating in the only project that matters.

We are cleansing that shiny stuff—the stuff of our selves and of the world that reflects our beliefs back into our own eyes—off the mirror that surrounds us. Because what's on the other side of that mirror is what's real.

It's your birthright, your heritage, and your destiny. You'll experience it again when you depart, just as you did before you arrived. You won't just experience it—you'll be it.

Why not get a head start?

CHAPTER 27

The Ultimate Choice

Your time has come. You've been through the horror of your cancer diagnosis, the ordeal of the workup and treatment, the anxiety that comes when they tell you your treatment is finished. You can't stop wondering if that's really true.

After a few months of uncertainty, those dreaded symptoms return. Your doctors tell you what you need to go through next. There's a new immunotherapy drug. You try it, and it buys more time. Then the symptoms recur. You're back to ground zero.

You've arrived at the place that all patients dread. No more treatments are available. Your doctors say those words that should never be uttered: *There's nothing more we can do.*

That's a lie, but you don't know it yet.

You think you're out of options. You feel abandoned and bereft. You experience the purity of pure despair. You are facing death.

Although you may feel certain that no one could possibly grasp the enormity of your distress, that's not true. Every single human being who has lived on this earth has faced what you are now facing—or they will in a future that is approaching faster than they might like.

You may believe you have no more options, but you do have a choice. The odds of curing your disease may be low, but a warehouse of opportunities for your healing has been unsealed.

Experienced and accomplished healers may be no further away from you than the phone in your hand. Palliative care and hospice people are well acquainted with the dread you feel, and they have a lot of practice at relieving it, along with the pain and other complaints that may be nagging you.

After you meet them, you start to feel some relief. You wonder why no one introduced these people to you before.

But your opportunities are still not exhausted. You have one more choice to make. And you don't have to wait until your body ceases to exist to make the ultimate choice: to let your self cease to exist. Even if this happens only for a moment, you have touched the eternal.

You may be one of the fortunate few who made this choice years before you were forced by illness to confront it. But whatever you have decided in the past, it's never too late to make the ultimate choice.

The ultimate decision is to surrender: to trust that this single precious, present moment you experience in pure consciousness is your own personal eternity. You may be surprised to discover that this moment and the next, and the one after that, are filled with a peace that surpasses your understanding.

Many who have gone before you have made this same decision: to let go and to simply trust. To surrender into the discovery that you are already cared for, now and through eternity.

The ultimate choice is to surrender your self so that only the real *you* remains.

May peace endure through all your moments here.

Acknowledgments

This book is dedicated to my wife and partner Barbara, but that's not enough. Unlike me, she doesn't have to work at being spiritual. She's already connected. She saw right through me the first moment we met. She always notices when my wounded self pulls me off course, and she helps line me up again. She's usually very kind when she does this, unless I need a little roughing up. Life will sand off your rough edges if you let it. I'm lucky to have such a highly skilled finish carpenter.

Many thanks to my kids, Carly and Jonah, who had to put up with my insane on-call work hours and my crazy ideas when they were young. Then Ingo came on board along with Barbara, and he's been just as patient with me. Now our three kids are scattered over the Western world with children of their own. We must have done something right as parents because they all know how to laugh, especially at their dad.

This book has been almost fifty years in the making. It might never have been written without the help and support of Christine Kloser and the team at Capucia Publishing. They encourage authors to write books about transformation. They mention in passing that the writing will transform the author. You have no idea. In particular, I want to thank my editor Karen Burton. More than a collaborator, she's a fellow spiritual traveler.

My late (and ex-) father-in-law, Willis Harman, helped set me on the path of discovery that led to the writing of this book. Not only was he the president of the Institute of Noetic Sciences when I was close with him, but he was also a psychedelic pioneer. I wish he were alive today to witness the renaissance in their research. To top it all off, he played a mean trombone.

Two men helped me find my way through my own personal darkness and out the other side. David Morgenstern saw who I was, and more importantly, who I could be. Michael Whitson held the faith for me when I'd lost the will to do it myself.

Khue Nguyen brings visions down to earth and makes them work in the world. Her spiritual heritage has facilitated healthcare transformation across the U.S. I'll always value our deep conversations that made cross-country flights go by in an instant.

Finally, I'm calling out my buds, the Drexel Misfits. We lived together half a century ago through a time in American history that left its imprint on all of us. None of us knows how long we have left, but navigating through our lives together today somehow makes that fact a little more manageable.

References

Abbey, Edward. 2015. *A Voice Crying in the Wilderness: Vox Clamantis in Deserto*. New York: Rosetta Books.

Barrett, Frederick S., Matthew W. Johnson, and Roland R. Griffiths. 2015. "Validation of the Revised Mystical Experience Questionnaire in experimental sessions with psilocybin." *Journal of Psychopharmacology*. October. doi: 10.1177/0269881115609019

Becker, Ernest. 2007. *The Denial of Death*. New York: Simon & Schuster.

Brewer, Judson A., Patrick J. Worhunsky, and Jeremy R. Gray. 2011. "Meditation experience is associated with differences in default mode network activity and connectivity." *Proceedings of the National Academy of Sciences (PNAS)*. 23 November. doi/full/10.1073/pnas.1112029108

Carhartt-Harris, Robin L., and Karl J. Friston. 2010. "The default mode, ego functions and free energy: A neurobiological account of Freudian ideas." *Brain*. April. pubmed.ncbi.nlm.nih.gov/20194141/

Carhartt-Harris, Robin L., David Erritzoe, Tim Williams, and David J. Nutt. 2012. "Neural correlates of the psychedelic state as determined by fMRI studies with psilocybin." *Proceedings of the National Academy of Science (PNAS)*. 23 January. doi.org/10.1073/pnas.1119598109

Chalmers, David. 2007. "The hard problem of consciousness." *The Blackwell Companion to Consciousness*. Hoboken, NJ: Blackwell Publishing, Ltd. eclass.uoa.gr/modules/document/file.php/PHS360/chalmers%20 The%20Hard%20Problem%20of%20consciousness.pdf

Chesterton, G. K. 1908. *Orthodoxy*. San Francisco: Ignatius Press.

Chi, Tingying and Jessica A. Gold. 2020. "A review of emerging therapeutic potential of psychedelic drugs in the treatment of psychiatric illnesses." *Journal of Neurological Science*. April 15. doi: 10.1016/j.jns.2020.116715

Clark, Maryam. 2022. "A replay of life: What happens in our brain when we die?" *Frontiers Science News*. 22 February. blog.frontiersin. org/2022/02/22/what-happens-in-our-brain-when-we-die/

Craig, Anne. 2022. "Discovery of 'thought worms' opens window to the mind." *Queens Gazette*: *Queens University*. 19 October. queensu. ca/gazette/stories/discovery-thought-worms-opens-window-mind

Flynn, Tom. 2002. "Secular Humanism Defined." *Free Inquiry*. Summer. secularhumanism.org/what-is-secular-humanism/secular-humanism-defined/

Fogel, Alan. 2021. "Restorative Embodied Self-Awareness." *Psychology Today*. 30 August. psychologytoday.com/us/blog/body-sense/202108/ restorative-embodied-self-awareness_

Friston, Karl. 2010. "The free-energy principle: A unified brain theory?" *Nature Reviews Neuroscience*. 13 January. nature.com/articles/nrn2787

Früh, Anton, et al. 2021. "Catalase Predicts In-Hospital Mortality after Out-of-Hospital Cardiac Arrest." *Journal of Clinical Medicine*. 30 August 2021. ncbi.nlm.nih.gov/pmc/articles/PMC8432041/

Goff, Philip. 2019. *Galileo's Error: Foundations of a New Science of Consciousness.* New York: Pantheon Books.

Goodwin, Guy M., et al. 2022. "Single-Dose Psilocybin for a Treatment-Resistant Episode of Major Depression." *New England Journal of Medicine.* 3 November. doi:10.1056/NEJMoa2206443

Griffiths, Roland R., et al. 2018. "Psilocybin-occasioned mystical-type experience in combination with meditation and other spiritual practices produces enduring positive changes in psychological functioning and in trait measures of prosocial attitudes and behaviors." *Journal of Psychopharmacology.* Jan. pubmed.ncbi.nlm.nih.gov/29020861/

Grof, Stanislav. 2008. *LSD Psychotherapy.* Santa Cruz, CA: Multidisciplinary Association for Psychedelic Studies.

Groves, James E. 1978. "Taking Care of the Hateful Patient." *New England Journal of Medicine.* 298(16) 883–887. May. doi:10.1056/NEJM197804202981605

Gusnard, Deborah A., Erbil Akbudak, Gordon L. Shulman, and Marcus E. Raichle. 2001. "Medial prefrontal cortex and self-referential mental activity: Relation to a default mode of brain function." *Proceedings of the National Academy of Sciences.* 20 March. doi.org/10.1073/pnas.071043098

Holze, Friederika, et al. 2022. "Direct comparison of the acute effects of lysergic acid diethylamide with psilocybin in a double-blind placebo-controlled study in healthy subjects." *Neuropsychopharmacology.* 25 February. nature.com/articles/s41386-022-01297-2

Huxley, Aldous. 2009. *The Doors of Perception and Heaven and Hell.* New York: Harper Perennial Modern Classic.

Kastrup, Bernardo. 2018. "Coming to Grips with the Implications of Quantum Mechanics." *Scientific American.* 29 May. blogs. scientificamerican.com/observations/coming-to-grips-with-the-implications-of-quantum-mechanics/

Kastrup Bernardo. 2019. *The Idea of the World: A Multi-Disciplinary Argument for the Mental Nature of Reality.* Washington: Iff Books.

Killingsworth, Matthew A. and Daniel T. Gilbert. 2010. "A Wandering Mind Is an Unhappy Mind." *Science.* 12 November. doi:10.1126/science.1192439

Krebs, Terri S. and Pal-Orjan Johansen. 2013. "Over 30 million psychedelic users in the United States." *F1000 Research.* 28 March. doi: 10.12688/f1000research.2-98.v1

Lao Tsu. *Tao Te Ching.* 2012. New York: Vintage Books.

Mack, Katie. 2020. *The End of Everything (Astrophysically Speaking).* New York: Scribner.

McNamara, Patrick. 2021. "Rem Sleep, the Default Mode Network and Behavioral Modernity." *Psychology Today.* 12 July. psychologytoday. com/us/blog/dream-catcher/202107/rem-sleep-the-default-mode-network-and-behavioral-modernity

Moody, Raymond. 1975. *Life After Life.* New York: Harper Collins.

Nagel, Thomas. 1974. "What is it like to be a bat?" *The Philosophical Review.* 83(4):435-450. doi:10.2307/2183914.

Nayda, Diane M. And Melanie KT Takarangi. 2021."The cost of being absent: Is meta-awareness of mind-wandering related to depression symptom severity, rumination tendencies and trauma intrusions?" *Journal of Affective Disorders.* 01 September. doi.org/10.1016/j. jad.2021.05.053

Nichols, David E. 2016. "Psychedelics." *Pharmacological Reviews*. April. doi.org/10.1124/pr.115.011478

Nichols, David E., et al. 2016. "Psychedelics as Medicines: An Emerging New Paradigm." *American Society for Clinical Pharmacology & Therapeutics*. 04 November. ascpt.onlinelibrary.wiley.com/doi/abs/10.1002/cpt.557

Nimbalkar, Namita. 2011. "John Locke on Personal Identity." *Mens Sana Monographs*. Jan–Dec; 9(1): 268–275. doi: 10.4103/0973-1229.77443

Parnia, Sam, et al. 2022. "Guidelines and standards for the study of death and recalled experiences of death—a multidisciplinary consensus statement and proposed future directions." *The New York Academy of Sciences*. 18 February. doi.org/10.1111/nyas.14740

Pew Research Center. 2022. "Frequency of Meditation." *Religious Landscape Study*, *Pew Research Center*. pewresearch.org/religion/religious-landscape-study/frequency-of-meditation/#demographic-information

Prinzig, Michael, Patty Van Kapellen, and Barbara L. Frederickson. 2021. "More than a Momentary Blip in the Universe? Investigating the Link Between Religiousness and Perceived Meaning in Life." *Personality and Social Psychology Bulletin*. 29 December. doi.org/10.1177/01461672211060136

Pueyo, Tomas. 2022. "The Ineluctable Progress of English." *Uncharted Territories*. 05 February. unchartedterritories.tomaspueyo.com/p/the-ineluctable-progress-of-english

Raichle, Marcus E. 1998. "The neural correlates of consciousness: An analysis of cognitive skill learning." *Philosophical Transactions of the Royal Society B*. 20 November. doi: 10.1098/rstb.1998.0341

Raichle, Marcus E. 2015. "The brain's default mode network." *Annual Review of Neuroscience*. 8 July. 38:433–447. doi: 10.1146/annurev-neuro-071013-014030

Ross, Stephen, et al. 2016. "Rapid and sustained symptom reduction following psilocybin treatment for anxiety and depression in life-threatening cancer: A randomized controlled trial." *Journal of Psychopharmacology*. 30(12):1165–1180, December. doi:10.1177/0269881116675512

Ross, Stephen, et al. 2021. "Acute and Sustained Reductions in Loss of Meaning and Suicidal Ideation Following Psilocybin-Assisted Psychotherapy for Psychiatric and Existential Distress in Life-Threatening Cancer." *American Cancer Society Pharmacology and Translational Science*. 18 March. doi.org/10.1021/acsptsci.1c00020

Rovelli, Carlo. 2021. "Quantum weirdness isn't weird—if we accept objects don't exist." *New Scientist*. 10 March. newscientist.com/article/mg24933250-500-quantum-weirdness-isnt-weird-if-we-accept-objects-dont-exist/

Rovelli, Carlo. 2021. *Helgoland: Making Sense of the Quantum Revolution.* New York: Riverhead Books.

Siegel, Ethan. 2021. "What does Einstein's General Relativity Actually Mean?" *Starts with a Bang.* 22 September. medium.com/starts-with-a-bang/what-does-einsteins-general-relativity-actually-mean-d185ebd287e0

Siegel, Ethan. 2022. "Ask Ethan: Did our Universe really arise from nothing?" *Starts with a Bang.* 04 March. bigthink.com/starts-with-a-bang/universe-nothing

Singer, Michael A. 2007. *The Untethered Soul: The Journey Beyond Yourself.* Oakland, CA: New Harbinger Publications, Inc.

Smigielski, Lukasz, Milan Scheidegger, Michael Kometer, and Franz X. Vollenweider. 2019. "Psilocybin-assisted mindfulness training modulates self-consciousness and brain default mode network connectivity with lasting effects." *NeuroImage.* 01 August. doi. org/10.1016/j.neuroimage.2019.04.009

Taylor, Jill Bolte. 2008. *My Stroke of Insight: A Brain Scientist's Personal Journey.* New York, NY: Viking Books.

Tolle, Eckhart. 1999. *The Power of Now: A Guide to Spiritual Enlightenment.* Novato, CA: New World Library.

Trimble, Michael R. 2013. *The Soul in the Brain: The Cerebral Basis of Language, Art, and Belief.* Baltimore, MD: Johns Hopkins University Press.

Urban, Tim. 2014. "What Makes You You?" *Wait But Why.* 12 December. waitbutwhy.com/2014/12/what-makes-you-you.html

van Elk, Michiel, et al. 2019. "The neural correlates of the awe experience: Reduced default mode network activity during feelings of awe." *Human Brain Mapping.* 15 August. doi: 10.1002/hbm.24616

Vicente, Raul, et al. 2022. "Enhanced Interplay of Neuronal Coherence and Coupling in the Dying Human Brain." *Frontiers in Aging Neuroscience.* 22 February. frontiersin.org/articles/10.3389/fnagi.2022.813531/full

Watts, Rosalind, et al. 2017. "Patients' Accounts of Increased 'Connectedness' and 'Acceptance' After Psilocybin Therapy for Treatment-Resistant Depression." *Journal of Humanistic Psychology.* 19 June. doi.org/10.1177/0022167817709585

Weinberg, Stephen. 1977. *The First 3 Minutes: A Modern View of the Origin of the Universe.* New York: Perseus Books.

About the Author

Brad Stuart, MD, practiced general internal medicine, treating patients in his office, the emergency room, the hospital, and the ICU. The latter half of his career was devoted to care of the dying. He first served as a hospice medical director in 1993 and later became Chief Medical Director for hospice services at the largest not-for-profit healthcare system in Northern California.

In the mid-1990s, he headed a team that worked with the National Hospice and Palliative Care Organization to develop national guidelines for hospice eligibility in non-cancer disease. In the early 2000s, he was the architect of the Advanced Illness Management (AIM) program, which won a $13 million grant from the Centers for Medicare and Medicaid Innovation and became a foundational element of new payment models developed by Medicare for the care of seriously ill patients and their families at home.

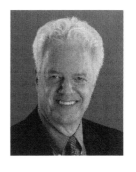

Dr. Stuart has written over fifty peer-reviewed papers and book chapters. He has given hundreds of talks internationally on clinical, emotional, and spiritual issues faced by people who are seriously ill and their loved ones.

He has three children and five grandchildren scattered across Oregon, Washington, DC, and Germany. He lives in Sonoma County, California, among the redwoods with his wife Barbara and a pond full of happy koi fish.

Made in United States
Troutdale, OR
08/31/2023